THE WAKING BRAIN

(Second Edition, Third Printing)

THE WAKING BRAIN

By

H. W. MAGOUN, Ph.D.

Brain Research Institute and Department of Anatomy
University of California at Los Angeles

Veterans Administration Hospital
Long Beach, California

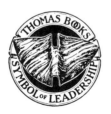

CHARLES C THOMAS • PUBLISHER
Springfield • Illinois • U.S.A.

Published and Distributed Throughout the World by
CHARLES C THOMAS • PUBLISHER
BANNERSTONE HOUSE
301-327 East Lawrence Avenue, Springfield, Illinois, U.S.A.
NATCHEZ PLANTATION HOUSE
735 North Atlantic Boulevard, Fort Lauderdale, Florida, U.S.A.

First Edition, First Printing, 1958
First Edition, Second Printing, 1960
Second Edition, 1963
Second Edition, Second Printing, 1964
Second Edition, Third Printing, 1965

With THOMAS BOOKS *careful attention is given to all details of
manufacturing and design. It is the Publisher's desire to present books
that are satisfactory as to their physical qualities and artistic possibilities
and appropriate for their particular use.* THOMAS BOOKS *will be true
to those laws of quality that assure a good name and good will.*

Printed in the United States of America

D-1

ACKNOWLEDGMENTS

Grateful acknowledgment is expressed for grants to the University of California from the Commonwealth Fund, the National Institutes of Health and the Ford Foundation, which have made possible much of the work of the Los Angeles group reported here.

CONTENTS

	Page
Acknowledgments	v

Chapter

1. HISTORICAL INTRODUCTION 3
2. RETICULO-SPINAL INFLUENCES AND POSTURAL REGULATION 23
   Facilitation and Inhibition 23
   Spasticity 24
   Nature of Inhibition 28
   Reticulo-spinal Action 31
   Gamma Efferents and Muscle Spindle Regulation 33
3. RETICULO-HYPOTHALAMIC INFLUENCES UPON ENDOCRINE AND
   VISCERAL FUNCTIONS 39
   Regulation of Pituitary-adrenocortical Activity 40
   Gastrointestinal and Cardiovascular Pathology 41
   Regulation of Pituitary-thyroid Activity 45
   Regulation of Pituitary-gonadal Activity 46
4. LIMBIC SYSTEMS FOR INNATE AND EMOTIONAL BEHAVIOR 53
   Innate Behavior 54
   Alimentary Behavior 55
   Mating Behavior 59
   Positive and Negative Reinforcement 59
   Aggressive Behavior 63
   Amygdala 65
   Forebrain and Inhibition of Behavior 68
5. RETICULO-CORTICAL INFLUENCES FOR WAKEFULNESS,
   ORIENTING AND ATTENTION 74
   Classic Contributions 74
   Ascending Reticular System 76
   Afferent Connections with the Reticular Formation 81
   Reticular System and the Anesthetic State 85

Page

Specificity Within the Non-specific System............. 87
Relation to Pain System........................... 87
Cortical Changes in EEG Arousal.................... 88

6. CORTICO-RETICULAR RELATIONS 98
Centrifugal Control of Afferent Function.............. 100
Afferent Conduction During Focus of Attention........ 103
Habituation 106
Sensory Deprivation 108
Orienting Reflex 109
External Inhibition 112

7. CONTRIBUTIONS TO THE ELECTROPHYSIOLOGY OF LEARNING... 116
Electrocortical Conditioning 116
Influence of Reinforcement in Learning................ 121
Physiological Architecture of the Conditional Reflex.... 124

8. PROCESSING OF INFORMATION INTO MEMORY.............. 129
Korsakoff's Syndrome 132
Experimental Temporal Lobectomy.................. 133
Hippocampal Theta Rhythm....................... 135
Neuroglial Function 140
Electron Microscopy of Glial-neuronal Relations........ 143
RNA and Memory................................ 148

9. BRAIN MECHANISMS FOR INTERNAL INHIBITION AND LIGHT
SLEEP 158
Thalamo-cortical Mechanisms for Internal Inhibition.... 159
Bulbar Driving of Thalamo-cortical System............ 161
Satiety and Internal Inhibition...................... 162
Caudate Driving of Thalamo-cortical System........... 169
Internal Inhibition of Higher Nervous Activity.......... 170

10. DEEP SLEEP 178
Differentiation of Light and Deep Sleep............... 178
Pontile Mechanism for Deep Sleep................... 181
General Features of Light and Deep Sleep............. 183

11. CONCLUSION 187

THE WAKING BRAIN

1

HISTORICAL INTRODUCTION

Wʜᴇɴ ᴏɴᴇ ʜᴀs sᴜʀᴠɪᴠᴇᴅ more than half a century, it becomes of interest to compare points of view at the beginning of such a period with those in which one's interest and activity are currently channeled. Besides the satisfaction which this may yield if it can be made to suggest that work with which one has been associated has contributed in some degree toward advancing knowledge, such a pursuit may possess the additional value of suggesting that one's investment of enthusiasm should not at any stage gain too great rigidity for, in another half-century or before, it is likely to be necessary to point out how inadequate currently accepted outlooks have become.

CONTEMPORARY BACKGROUND

The period of the turn of the century, called Edwardian for its coincidence with the reign of Edward VII, saw the beginning of modern developments in the physiology of the central nervous system. The contributions to an understanding of reflex function and developments in the field of cortical localization represented the two great advances of this period. This progress built upon the accomplishments in study of peripheral nerve and receptors in the just preceding latter half of the nineteenth century.

The tendency to sharp categorization of activities which marked these achievements was a feature characterizing the Edwardian era generally. The reflex arc lent itself to the clear-cut distinction of an afferent and an efferent limb. Its fundamental arc was re-elaborated in a higher elevation, to and from precisely organized sensory and motor areas of the cortex, in which elaborate somatotopic representation possessed all the formal order and pattern so typical of the Edwardian world. At the segmental level, the reflex arc was proposed to provide the neural basis for

[3]

simple adjustive activity, proceeding in an involuntary manner; while its more elevated reflexion, the sensori-motor arc through the cortex served subjective perception and voluntary motion. Provision thus seemed at hand for understanding our sensory appreciation of the external world, as well as accounting for our involuntary and willed performance in it, in terms of super-imposed levels of neural organization and complexity.

A long series of earlier developments preceded this brilliant synthesis of the Edwardian period, for it is remarkable how early and how generally in history man sought to systematize and to refer focally, his capacities to perceive and move, to feel and behave, to develop relations with his fellow-man—and with woman, to hope, plan, labor and, occasionally, to achieve.

PLATONIC SOUL

The brain, "which some suppose the soul's frail dwelling-house," had initially to compete seriously with other organs as the seat of the faculties. In Greek antiquity, Plato (Cornford, 1952) and Aristotle (Hicks, 1907) advanced the head and the heart, respectively, as the chief contending sites; and, in the seventeenth century, the question still was asked, "Tell me, where is fancy bred—or in the heart or in the head" (Shakespeare). Plato's tripartite soul, the properties of which corresponded to some degree with those of plant, animal, and man, was given serial representation in the major cavities of the body (Fig. 1, left). The vegetative soul, serving appetite and nutrition, was placed lowest in the pelvis and belly; the vital soul, responsible for body heat, was next above in the chest; while the crowning, rational soul fittingly occupied the highest elevation in the head. In later elaboration, the activities of these souls were conceived to be managed by three matching spirits, initially derived from in-gested food, in the liver; transmuted, with inspired air, in the heart; to gain their most advanced perfection in the cranium, as animal (psychic) spirits serving the functions of the brain.

HYDRAULIC MODEL

Each period in succession sought a relevant physical model of vital phenomena; and the brain, in particular, has been

likened to the most complex analogue of each age. The Galenic
synthesis of classical neurobiology drew naturally upon the reser-
voirs, aqueducts, fountains, baths and sewers of the Greco-
Roman period, some of which are still preserved, in conceiving
of neural function in hydraulic terms. The three-chambered
cerebral ventricles were recognized from Alexandrian times (Fig.
1, right), and a partial transverse division of the brain by the
tentorium was stressed by Galen (May, 1956) as separating a
soft, sensory part, before; from a hard, motor one, behind (Fig. 2,
left). Succeeding Islamic and mediaeval scholars elaborated an
orderly spatial distribution of the faculties in relation to this
plan (Magoun, 1958).

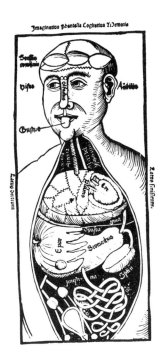
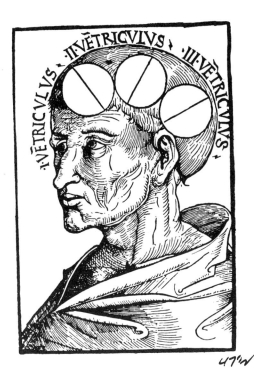

Fig. 1. (*Left*) Anatomical figure from Peyligk (1518), showing the divi-
sions of the body into the head, chest, belly and pelvis. Note the ventricles
in the brain, with their faculties labeled above. (*Right*) The three ventricular chambers in the head, from an early printed edition of Albertus Magnus
(1506).

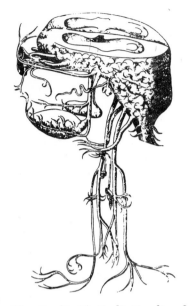 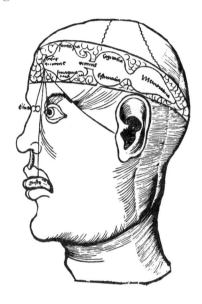

Fig. 2. (*Left*) Early Vesalian figure, showing the Galenic division of the brain into an anterior part, to which the sensory nerves are attached; and a posterior part, from which the motor nerves emerge. From Choulant (1920). (*Right*) Early printed woodcut, showing the reference of the faculties to the ventricular chambers of the brain. From Reisch (1504).

Respecting Galen's views, information was gathered from various receptors and interrelated in the *sensus communis* in the anterior cerebral cavities (Fig. 2, right). Integrative activities, including judgment, cogitation and estimation, proceeded in the middle ventricle. Both memory and motion were seated in the posterior chamber, in relation to which the efferent nerves arose; for the hard nature of the posttentorial brain, proposed by Galen on a motor basis, further insured that an impression once made here would not easily be erased. This sequential reference of sensory, integrative and motor faculties, from the front to the back of the head, conveyed an implication that neural activities normally proceeded through these stages, familiar to us today.

DIOPTRICAL MODEL

In the seventeenth and eighteenth centuries, more dynamic analogies between mechanical automata and living bodies developed from advances in the physical sciences. Relating his own studies of geometry and dioptrics to the brain, Descartes (1677) conceived that, as the spirits reached the ventricular cavities, they were reflected like rays of light to appropriate motor channels (Fig. 3, left). Special significance was attached to the pineal body, the unpaired nature of which, familiar to Descartes from dissection, permitted synthesis of information from the two halves of the body, just as its median position made possible the initiation of movement bilaterally and equivalently in all directions. Additionally, and possibly from the importance attached to valves in Harvey's discovery of the circulation of the blood, Descartes conceived of the pineal as a valvular mechanism which, by inclination from a neutral position, could influence the course of the spirits between the cerebral ventricles and the pores of the nerves which lined their walls (Fig. 3, right). More generally, he urged that the functions of the brain should be considered "as following altogether naturally, in this machine, from the disposition of its parts alone, neither more nor less than do the movements of a clock or other automaton." Following Descartes, stereotype responses became explicable in mechanical terms and derived, from his description of the *reflection* of spirits, their designation, *reflex* (Fearing, 1929).

PHRENOLOGICAL MODEL

Attention next became directed to the cerebral hemispheres, the cortex of which was observed to increase progressively through the animal series, to reach its greatest development in man. The higher faculties then seemed more logically to have their reference here, than in older and phylogenetically more stable structures, bordering the deep-lying ventricles of the brain. In the first, irresponsible, romantic half of the nineteenth century, Gall and Spurzheim (Ackerknecht and Vallois, 1956) parcellated man's psychological faculties over the surface of these hemispheres, the unusual development of a faculty being attributed to regional cortical hypertrophy, leading, in turn, to a local bulging of the overlying cranium. Consequent exploration of the bumps of the head, it was proposed, might provide insight into an individual's personality and reveal his unsuspected abilities.

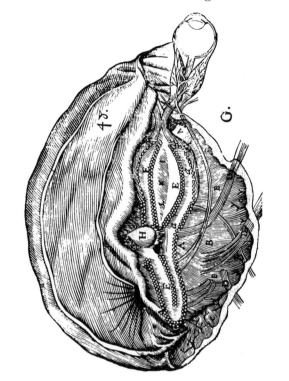

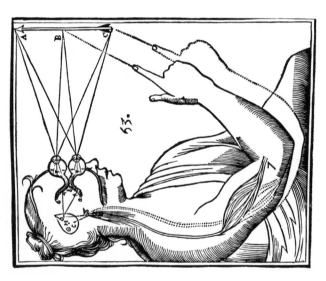

Fig. 3. (*Left*) The first diagram of the reflex arc, from Descartes' *Treatise on Man* (1677). Like rays of light, spirits from the pores of the optic nerves are *reflected* from the pineal body (H) to the pores of the motor nerves, so as to induce a response appropriate to the stimulus. (*Right*) Figure from Descartes' *Treatise on Man* (1677), showing the brain ventricles lined by the pores of the nerves. The central pineal body (H) is strategically located to influence the course of the spirits within the ventricular chambers.

In that period, such phrenological examination aroused widespread popular interest, comparable perhaps to that of psychological testing today.

GEOLOGICAL MODEL

In the second, more sober, scientific half of the nineteenth century, thinking was dominated by concepts of evolution, first of the earth and then of living things and man. Following Lyell (1834) and Darwin (1859), development of the brain came to be explained by the addition in phylogeny of a succession of neural levels, with each higher increment serving more complex functions and dominating over those below (Fig. 4). In sketches of an invertebrate ganglion, Herbert Spencer (1855) showed how a neural plexus could adjust to increased environmental demands by the successive addition of higher coordinating layers which, of necessity, were protuberant and superimposed because

ENGLISH NEUROLOGY Hughlings Jackson	RUSSIAN NEUROPHYSIOLOGY Ivan P. Pavlov	COMPARATIVE NEUROANATOMY Edinger, Kappers, Herrick	PSYCHOANALYTIC PSYCHIATRY Sigmund Freud	SYNTHESIS
HIGHEST LEVEL	SECOND SIGNAL SYSTEM		SUPER EGO	ABSTRACTION DISCRIMINATION SYMBOLIZATION COMMUNICATION
MIDDLE LEVEL	CONDITIONED REFLEX		EGO	ACQUIRED ADAPTIVE BEHAVIOR
LOWEST LEVEL	UNCONDITIONED REFLEXES		ID	INNATE STEREOTYPED PERFORMANCE

Fig. 4. Chart comparing the evolutionary concepts of organization and function of the brain which developed after Darwin and Spencer. From Magoun (1960).

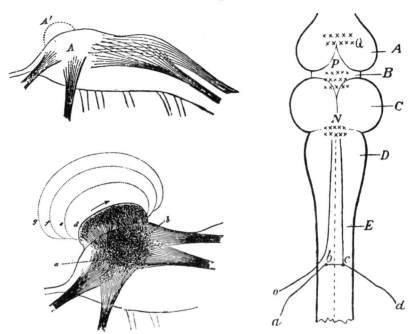

Fig. 5. (*Left*) Diagrams of invertebrate ganglion, prepared by Spencer (1855), showing the manner of development of superimposed levels of neural coordination. (*Right*) Diagram of the central nervous system of the frog, from Sechenov (1935). Stimulation of the sites marked by crosses inhibited spinal reflexes, illustrating the hierarchy of neural levels and the dominance of higher over those below.

of the preemption of the original space (Fig. 5, left). Shortly thereafter, Sechenov (1863) extended this concept to the vertebrate nervous system, when he stimulated the brain of the frog by applying crystals of salt to its surface. At brain stem sites (Fig. 5, right), such excitation slowed or prevented the activity of spinal reflexes and, in these seminal experiments, the father of Russian physiology provided evidence for a hierarchy of levels, with the higher dominating over those below and, incidentally, discovered central neural inhibition.

The full elaboration of this geological model of the brain was primarily a post-Darwinian development, however. Contributory figures included Hughlings Jackson (1958) in neurology, Edinger (1885) in comparative anatomy, Pavlov (1955) in physiology and Freud (1954) in psychiatry. In each case, management of the internal environment of the body, as well as innate behavior preserving the individual and the race, was attributed to older subcortical neural structures, forming Jackson's lowest level, and subserving Pavlov's unconditional reflexes and the Freudian *Id* (Fig. 6). Next, the more mutable, adaptive, learned performance of conditional reflexes, together with the capacity of the *Ego* for perception and the initiation of movement, were attributed to the sensori-motor cortex, or Jackson's middle level, which developed above or upon the older subjacent parts (Fig. 6). Finally, in the brain of man, increase of associational cortex, forming Jackson's highest level, provided among other things for Pavlov's second signal system, serving communication by spoken and written language, and for other cognitive, symbolic and discriminative functions, relating the individual to the external world and to his fellow man. In its progressive encephalization,

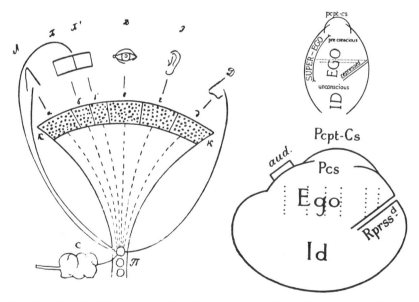

Fig. 6. (*Left*) Diagram of the Pavlovian conditional reflex (1955), by which adjustments to the environment are established through new links between the cortical analyzers and connections from them to subcortical unconditioned reflex arcs. (*Right*) Two diagrams by Freud (1954), presenting the mental apparatus as though spatially stratified.

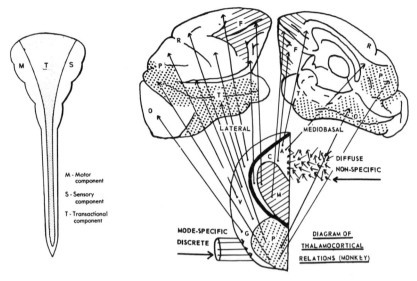

Fig. 7. (*Left*) A diagram showing the vertical organization of the nervous system, in terms of a central transactional core located between the more laterally placed and more differentiated sensory and motor components. From Livingston, Haugen and Brookhart (1954). (*Right*) Schematic representation of the differing cortical projections from the internal core and the external portion of the thalamus. The black band (below) indicates the division of the thalamus into an internal core, which receives a diffuse, nonspecific input; and an external portion, which receives discrete, modality-specific projection tracts. From Pribram (1958).

the brain thus came ultimately to resemble the earth itself, not simply in its globular form but in consisting as well of a series of horizontal strata laid down, like those of geology, one upon another through evolutionary time (Magoun, 1960).

EMBRYOLOGICAL MODEL

While phylogenetic approaches to evolution pointed to such an horizontal laminar plan, concurrent ontogenetic studies arrived at an orientation 90° out of phase and proposed, instead, a vertical organization of the brain. The embryologist, Karl Ernst von Baer (1837), advanced the principle of "progressive differentiation" when he wrote: "If one examines the progress of development, it is very conspicuous that from the homogeneous and the general, the heterogeneous and the special gradually emerge. With respect to the direction which such development takes, the observer notices at each moment that it proceeds from the center to the periphery. What there is first present of the embryo is clearly its middle, from which development proceeds to all sides."

Although the horizontal plan had gained wide support, occasional dissenters had appeared. On coming across von Baer's idea of progressive differentiation, Herbert Spencer (1862) was so strongly affected as to devote the balance of his career to its application to all fields of knowledge in a *System of Synthetic Philosophy*, contributions to which appeared throughout the latter part of the nineteenth century. Today, an increasing number of contemporary neural philosophers, Yakolev (1948), the elder Livingston (1954), Pribram (1958), Galambos (1959), and others have urged that fundamentally the adult as well as the embryonic central nervous system is vertically, rather than horizontally arranged (Fig. 7). As von Baer (1837) proposed, they point to the presence of older, more generalized core-components, developing first in ontogeny, in a central position close to the primitive neural tube, and go on to distinguish more specialized and differentiated structures, which have become added laterally as the nervous system matures.

TECHNOLOGICAL MODEL

Most recently, the mechanical materialism of the seventeenth and eighteenth centuries, with its analogies to clocks, and other automata, has swollen to a flood inundating all of biology and in particular the brain. Present concepts of neural organization and function propose models of self-adaptive automatic control mechanisms, derived from engineering and technology, and conceive of circular rather than vertical or horizontal arrangements of the brain.

Emphasis has been placed upon feedback, in which part of the output of an active system returns in a loop to modulate its continuing performance. When such feedback is positive, it provides a means of amplifying excursion or increasing performance. When negative, it provides a method of reducing the sys-

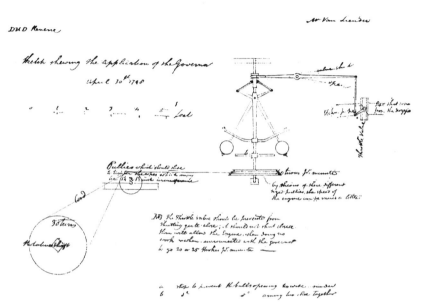

Fig. 8. Sketches of the governor contrived by Watt for automatic regulation of the speed of his steam engine. Two balls, revolving on hinged arms, play up and down a rod, rotating at engine speed. The centrifugal force of the balls' revolution governs the aperture of the throttle valve, which determines the passage of steam. When steam pressure is great and the tendency of the engine is to go faster, the governor reduces the steam; when it is less, the governor opens the throttle and increases the supply.
From Dickinson and Jenkins (1927).

tem's activity. Upon introduction of a device whereby the direction of each of these feedback influences becomes the inverse of that setting it into play, their alternate evocation tends to stabilize activity around an optimal level of performance and so preserves the homeostatic state (Fig. 8).

When such automatic control systems become disordered, unbalanced feedback influences swing performance increasingly wide of the mark, first in one direction and then the other, until a type of oscillation ensues. In the field of neurological disease, such spectacular symptoms as cerebellar ataxia, Parkinson's tremor, and the clonus of spastic hemiplegia all appear explicable in such terms. Less dramatic advances in histology and physiology have not attracted so much attention but have, nevertheless, contributed significantly to advancing concepts of neural organization and function in cybernetic terms.

In the hey-day of histology, Golgi (1959) described the recurrent axon-collateral of the large, type I neuron, together with the short-axoned, type II, internuncial cell (Fig. 9, left) and

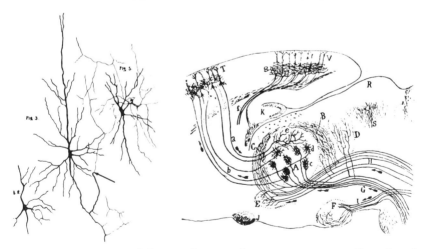

Fig. 9. (*Left*) Original figures showing the recurrent axon collateral and type II cell. From Golgi (1959).(*Right*) Ramon y Cajal's sketch of feedback organization of connections between the thalamus and cortex in the rodent brain (1952). In addition to ascending fibers (b) from the thalamus (A) to the cortex (T), Cajal described "descending sensory fibers" (a) from the cortex to the sensory thalamic nuclei and called these "fibres de l'attention expectante."

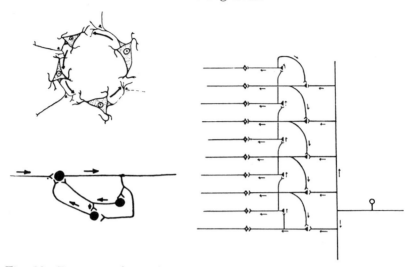

Fig. 10.   Diagrams of spinal neuronal circuits accounting for reflex after-discharge: *upper left,* from Kubie (1930); *lower left,* from Lorente de Nó (1933); *right,* from Ranson & Hinsey (1930).

Ramon y Cajal (1952) clearly identified cortico-thalamic feedbacks on microscopic grounds (Fig. 9, right). A half-century elapsed, however, before physiologists made conceptual use of Golgi's observations or explored Cajal's suggestion that "this mode of connection permits the cortex to act on specific areas of the sensory field, either to inhibit or to intensify activity."

In the nineteen twenties and thirties, attention was directed to reflex after-discharge which, in persisting after its evocative stimulus had ceased, was inexplicable in established S-R terms. In solution, Forbes (1922) postulated the recurrent bombardment of motoneurons by impulses arriving over progressively more complex "delay-paths." Because the supply of such long pathways seemed limited, advantage next was taken of Golgi's axon collaterals and short-axoned cells, and delay-paths were arranged in a circular, rather than linear order. Kubie (1930) (Fig. 10, upper left) and Lorente de Nó (1933) (Fig. 10, lower left) proposed "self-reexciting chains" of neurons; while Ranson and Hinsey (1930) advanced "reverberating circuits," in which closed rings of neurons were linked together by their axon collaterals (Fig. 10, right). Though no one did so in the thirties, it was possible to designate these neuronal circuits as positive feedbacks.

In a book entitled *Cybernetics or Control and Communication in the Animal and the Machine,* Wiener (1948) pointed out that "the present is truly the age of servo-mechanisms, as the nineteenth century was the age of the steam engine and the eighteenth the age of the clock." Grey Walter (1953) elaborated, in 1953: "With the coming of steam and later electricity, a new sort of automatic device became necessary to enable a machine to control its own effective use of the power it generates. The first steam engine, left to itself, was unstable—pressure went down when power was used and the boiler blew up when it was not. Watt (Dickinson and Jenkins, 1927) introduced the safety valve and automatic governor which stabilized by themselves both boiler pressure and engine speed (Fig. 8). These two important devices were taken rather as a matter of course by engineers, but the great Clerk Maxwell (1868) devoted a paper to the analysis of Watt's governor and was perhaps the first to realize the significance of this key process of feedback."

Having come then to the present day, it is possible to conclude this brief survey with the synthesis seen in Figure 11, in which concepts of neural organization are given graphic expression in their order of review. On the left are a series of horizontal levels, identified as the successive morphological segments of the brain. In the middle is a vertical arrangement, in which nonspecific systems are present in the central core, with more specific systems external to them. At the right, a series of recurrent loops provide for feedback control of postural, sensory, limbic and higher cortical functions. Happily, these models are supplementary rather than conflicting ones for, actually, the brain is organized in all these ways.

NONSPECIFIC RETICULAR SYSTEM

For our present purpose, earlier interest in the deep-lying ventricles and pineal body had the desirable feature of focusing attention upon the subcortical stem of the brain, a drawing of which, prepared by Sir Christopher Wren for Thomas Willis (1681), is shown in Figure 12. The labels, in Elizabethan Eng-

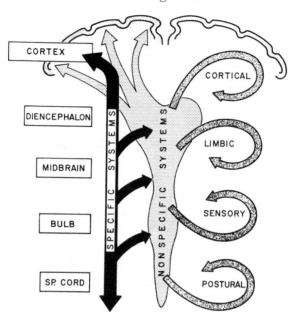

HORIZONTAL • VERTICAL • FEEDBACK

Fig. 11. Synthesis of horizontal (*left*), vertical (*center*) and circular (*right*) organization of the central nervous system. Modified by Galambos (1959).

lish, compare the mounds, protuberances, globular prominences and apertures of this region with familiar counterparts of perineal anatomy, suggesting that investigators of that age considered this region to be the literal *seat* of the soul. Full attention did not return to the brain stem until recently, however, for it will be recalled that Edwardian contributions to the physiology of the central nervous system were focused largely upon reflex functions of the spinal cord below and upon activities of the sensorimotor cortex above, leaving the intervening stem of the brain unattended.

Recent study has once more stressed the importance of this neural part, however, in identification of centrally placed, non-specific mechanisms, which parallel the more lateral, specific systems of classical neurology and are richly interconnected with

Tabu V

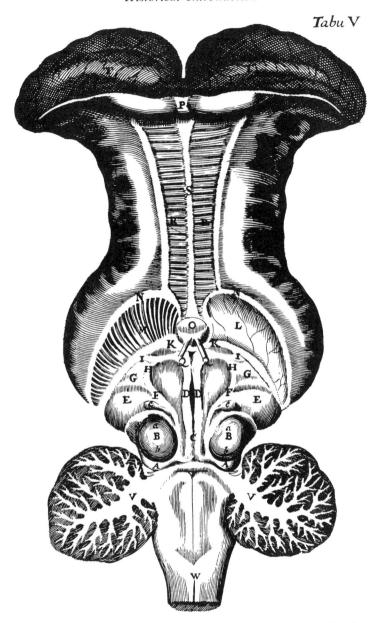

Fig. 12. Sheep brain "rolled forth to show the marrowy tracts" and provide a dorsal view of the brain stem. From Willis (1681).

them. These nonspecific mechanisms are distributed widely through the central core of the brain stem and, as spokes radiate from the hub of a wheel to its peripheral working rim, so functional influences of these central systems can be exerted in a number of directions: caudally upon spinal levels which influence postural and other activity; rostrally and ventrally upon hypothalamic and pituitary mechanisms, concerned with visceral and endocrine functions; cephalically upon the diencephalic and limbic brain, where affect and emotion now reign instead of in the heart; and more cephalically and dorsally still, upon the cortex of the cerebral hemispheres which, with its interconnected thalamic and basal ganglionic masses, serves all higher sensori-motor and intellectual performance.

Influences of these nonspecific systems in the brain stem are thus brought to bear upon most other portions and functions of the central nervous system, either to raise or to diminish the level of their activities or to integrate their several performances. Just as all spokes move together in the turning of a wheel, though they may bear weight sequentially, so the variously directed influences of these nonspecific reticular systems are closely interrelated in normal function (Brodal, 1957; French, 1958; Jasper, 1958; O'Leary and Cohen, 1958; Rossi and Zanchetti, 1957; Segundo, 1956). For purposes of presentation, they may be considered individually, however, and discussion may commence with reticular influences upon the spinal cord.

REFERENCES

Ackerknecht, E. H. and Vallois, H. V.: *Franz Joseph Gall, Inventor of Phrenology and his Collection.* Madison, University of Wisconsin Press, 1956.

Albertus Magnus: *Philosophia Naturalis.* Basel, 1506.

Baer, K. E.: *Über Entwickslungsgeschichte der Thiere.* Königsberg, 1837. Trans. by Bodemer, C., 1961.

Brodal, A.: *The Reticular Formation of the Brain Stem; Anatomical Aspects and Functional Correlations.* Oliver and Boyd, Edinburgh, 1957.

Choulant, L.: *History and Bibliography of Anatomic Illustration.* Trans. and ed. by Frank, M., University of Chicago Press, 1920.

Cornford, F. M.: *Plato's Cosmology, The Timaeus of Plato.* Trans. with running commentary. Humanities Press, New York, 1952.

Darwin, C.: *On the Origin of Species by Means of Natural Selection, or the Preservation of Favored Races in the Struggle for Life.* John Murray, London, 1859.

Descartes, R.: *L'homme de René Descartes.* Second ed., Paris, 1677. Trans. by Warwick, B., 1959.

Dickinson, H. W., and Jenkins, R.: *James Watt and the Steam Engine.* Clarendon Press, Oxford, 1927.

Edinger, L.: *Zehn Vorlesungen über den Bau der nervosen Zentralorgane.* Vogel, Leipzig, 1885.

Fearing, F.: René Descartes, a study in the history of the theories of reflex action. *Psychol. Rev.,* 36:375-388, 1929.

Forbes, A.: The interpretation of spinal reflexes in terms of present knowledge of nerve conduction. *Physiol. Rev.,* 2:361-414, 1922.

French, J. D.: The reticular formation. *J. Neurosurg.,* 15:97-115, 1958.

Freud, S.: *The Origins of Psycho-Analysis.* Basic Books, New York, 1954.

Galambos, R.: In Brazier, M. A. B. (Ed.) *The Central Nervous System and Behavior.* Macy Foundation, New York, 1959, pp. 288-290.

Golgi, C.: Recherches sur l'histologie des centres nerveuse. Reprinted, with historical review, by Fuortes, M.G.F. *Arch. Ital. Biol.,* 97:276-299, 1959.

Hicks, R. D.: *Aristotle, De Anima.* Cambridge University Press, Cambridge, 1907.

Jackson, J. H.: *Selected Writings of John Hughlings Jackson.* Two Vols. Basic Books, New York, 1958.

Jasper, H. H. (Ed.): *Reticular Formation of the Brain.* Little, Brown, Boston, 1958.

Kubie, L. S.: A theoretical application to some neurological problems of the properties of excitation waves which move in closed circuits. *Brain,* 53:166-177, 1930.

Livingston, W. K., Haugen, F. P. and Brookhart, J. M.: Functional organization of the central nervous system. *Neurology,* 4:485-496, 1954.

Lorente de Nó, R.: Vestibulo-ocular reflex arc. *Arch. Neurol. & Psychiat.,* 30:245-291, 1933.

Lyell, C.: *Principles of Geology.* John Murray, London, 1834.

Magoun, H. W.: Early development of ideas relating the mind with the brain. Ciba Foundation Symposium on the *Neurological Basis of Behavior.* 1958, Pp. 4-22.

Magoun, H. W.: Evolutionary concepts of brain function following Darwin and Spencer. In Tax, S.(Ed): *Evolution After Darwin.* University of Chicago Press, 1960.

Maxwell, J. C.: On governors. *Proc. Roy. Soc. London S.B.,* 16:270-283, 1868.

May, Mrs. F. A.: Galen's *De usu partium.* English translation (unpublished).

O'Leary, J. and Cohen, L. A.: The reticular core 1957. *Physiol. Rev.,* 38: 243-276, 1958.

Pavlov, I. P.: *Selected works.* Koshtoyants, K. S. (Ed) Foreign Languages Publishing House, Moscow, 1955.

Peyligk, J.: Compendiosa capitis physici declaratio (from *Philosophiae naturalis compendium*). Lipsi, imp. Wolfgangus Monacensis, 1518.

Pribram, K.: Comparative neurology and the evolution of behavior. In Roe, A. and Simpson, G. C. (Eds): *Behavior and Evolution.* Yale University Press, New Haven, 1958.

Ramon y Cajal, S.: Histologie du système nerveux. Vol. II. *Translated and reprinted from first Spanish edition (Vol. 1,* 1899; *Vol. 2,* 1904). Instituto Ramon y Cajal, Madrid, 1952.

Ranson, S. W. and Hinsey, J. C.: Reflexes in the hind limbs of cats after transection of the spinal cord at various levels. *Am. J. Physiol., 94:* 471-495, 1930.

Reisch, G.: *Margarita Philosophica. Argentori, per Joh. Grüninger,* 1504.

Rossi, G. R. and Zanchetti, A.: The brain stem reticular formation, anatomy and physiology. *Arch. Ital. Biol.,* 95:199-435, 1957.

Sechenov, I.: *Selected Works.* A. A. Subkov (Ed.) Moscow-Leningrad, 1935.

Segundo, J. P.: The reticular formation, a survey. *Acta Neurol. Latinoamer.,* 3:245-281, 1956.

Shakespeare, W.: *The Merchant of Venice.* Act III, Sc. 2, l. 63.

Spencer, H.: *Principles of Psychology.* Williams and Norgate. London, 1855.

Spencer, H.: *First Principles.* Williams and Norgate. London, 1862.

Walter, W. G.: *The Living Brain.* W. W. Norton. New York, 1953.

Wiener, N.: *Cybernetics or Control and Communication in the Animal and Machine.* Herman & Cie. Paris, 1948.

Willis, T.: *The Remaining Medical Works, etc.,* Englished by S. Pordage. London, 1681.

Yakolev, P. I.: Motility, behavior and the brain. *J. Nerv. & Ment. Dis.,* 107:313-335, 1948.

2

RETICULO-SPINAL INFLUENCES AND POSTURAL REGULATION

With growth of knowledge of the motor area of the cortex and its pyramidal pathway to spinal outflows, there developed also the concept of an extra-pyramidal motor mechanism concerned more with the coordination than with the initiation of movement. Its extra-pyramidal designation refers to pathways descending into the cord, outside the pyramidal tract, through the tegmentum and reticular formation of the brain stem. Except for the cortico-spinal tract, few if any fibers proceed directly from higher brain regions to the cord and, on anatomical grounds, intercalated reticulo-spinal connections form the major final common pathway of the extra-pyramidal motor system (Allen, 1932; Papez, 1926). Abundant support for this view has come from the influences upon motor activity which their excitation can induce (Magoun, 1950).

FACILITATION AND INHIBITION

Stimulation of different regions of the reticular formation can evoke powerful inhibition or facilitation of a wide range of motor performance including flexor and extensor reflexes, decerebrate rigidity, and cortical motor responses (Fig. 13). Under chloralosane or nembutal anesthesia, generalized effects are easily elicitable, and global inhibition or facilitation of spinal motor discharge can readily be induced (Fig. 14). Other work has stressed the reciprocal nature of reticulo-spinal influences, both upon antagonistic muscles acting at a given joint (Gernandt and Thulin, 1955) and upon symmetrical muscle groups on opposite halves of the body (Sprague and Chambers, 1954). A pattern of primitive progression, which combines reciprocal contraction of opposite limbs with a concavity of the spine, is in fact the

[23]

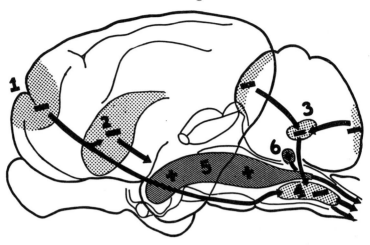

Fig. 13. Outline view of the brain of the cat showing facilitatory (5) and inhibitory (4) areas of the brain stem reticular formation and connections to the latter from the cerebral cortex (1) and cerebellum (3). From Lindsley, Schreiner and Magoun (1949).

only obtrusive result of reticular stimulation in the unanesthetized, behaving animal (Sprague and Chambers, 1954). Inability to evoke reticulo-spinal inhibition under these conditions may be attributable to negative feedback from the functioning cortex, reducing bulbar excitability, like that found by Hugelin and Bonvallet (1957) to reduce reticulo-spinal facilitation. In possible support, unimpaired reticulo-spinal inhibition and facilitation are both elicitable in the unanesthetized decerebrate preparation.

SPASTICITY

The inhibitory or facilitatory effects of reticular stimulation are exerted as markedly upon postural or stretch reflexes as upon phasic motor activity and, following chronic ablation of cerebellar and cortical regions which project to the reticular region, a pronounced exaggeration of stretch reflexes ensues (Magoun and Rhines, 1948; Lindsley, Schreiner and Magoun, 1949). With the passage of time, this initially marked and generalized stretch hyperreflexia becomes attenuated and limited to the anti-gravity musculature (Fig. 15). Excitability of the inhibitory component of the reticulo-spinal mechanism may be dependent upon bombardment by those cerebellar and cortical regions whose ablation is followed by spasticity and become deficient in their absence. Reduction or absence of this inhibitory reticulo-spinal influence would seem likely, by itself, to result in some exaggeration of spinal postural reflexes but the stretch hyperreflexia of spasticity appears to be determined by an important positive factor as well.

In animals with spasticity, succeeding transection of the thoracic spinal cord was followed by loss or marked reduction of exaggerated stretch reflexes in the lower extremity, the spinal innervation of which had been severed from the brain (Fig. 16). By contrast, myotatic reflexes in the upper extremity, whose spinal segments still remained connected with the brain, continued to be exaggerated. From this it appeared that the stretch hyperreflexia of spasticity should not be attributed solely to release from inhibition. The continued and unopposed presence of facilitation, conveyed by reticulo- and vestibulo-spinal connec-

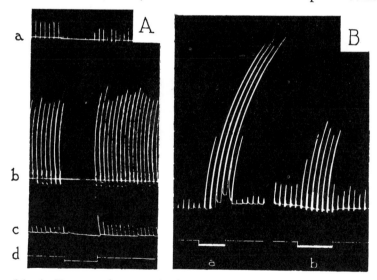

Fig. 14. A. Kymographic records showing inhibition of flexor (a), patellar (b) and blink (c) reflexes, during stimulation of bulbar reticular formation (signal). From Magoun and Rhines (1946). B. Increase of cortical motor response (a) and patellar reflex (b) during stimulation (signal) of facilitatory reticular area shown in Figure 13. From Rhines and Magoun (1946).

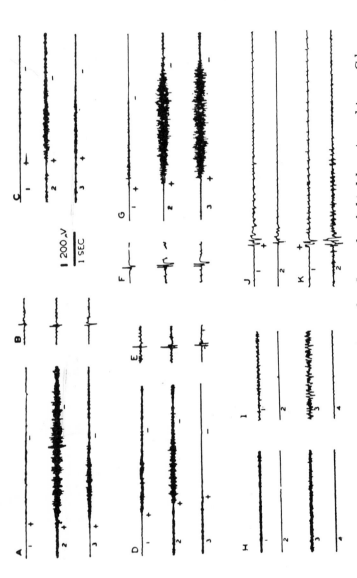

Fig. 15. Electromyographic records of stretch reflexes of cat's hind leg: A-quadriceps, C-hamstrings, D-tibialis and G-gastrocnemius, tested before (1) and four days (2) and one month (3) after combined lesions of pericruciate cortex, caudate and fastigial nuclei (see Fig. 13). Corresponding records of tendon jerks are shown: B-knee, E-tibialis and F-Achilles, the amplification of the preoperative records being twice that of the postoperative records. H, I-Levels of resting tension are present in quadriceps (1), and gastrocnemius (3), but not in hamstrings (2), or tibialis (3), ten days postoperatively. Clonus after Achilles jerk (J) and knee jerk (K) is seen postoperatively in gastrocnemius (1) and tibialis (2). From Lindsley, Schreiner and Magoun (1949).

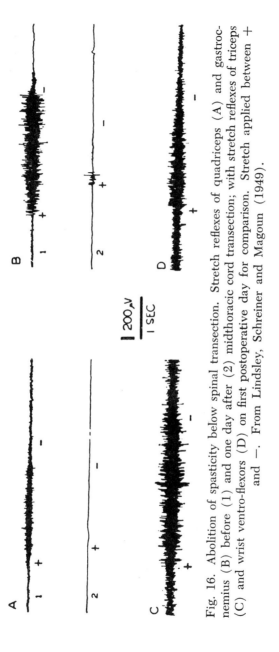

Fig. 16. Abolition of spasticity below spinal transection. Stretch reflexes of quadriceps (A) and gastroc-nemius (B) before (1) and one day after (2) midthoracic cord transection; with stretch reflexes of triceps (C) and wrist ventro-flexors (D) on first postoperative day for comparison. Stretch applied between + and —. From Lindsley, Schreiner and Magoun (1949).

tions from the brain, seems of additional importance and, for a time, spasticity may be secondarily abolished by its elimination.

In this respect, the behavior of the spinal stretch-reflex in spasticity resembles that of a Jack-in-the-box, who jumps up when the lid holding him down is removed. This simulated hyperactivity upon release, in which the charm of the Jack-in-the-box consists, can be shown to depend, moreover, both on the removal of a lid which holds him down and on a spring inside the box, which is the actual factor responsible for pushing him up. With current interest in mathematical expression in biology, it is possible to phrase the situation as an equation, involving—*one,* spinal stretch reflexes; *two,* inhibitory reticulo-spinal influences; and *three,* facilitatory reticulo-spinal influences—so that: *one,* minus *two,* plus *three,* equals spasticity. While these conclusions assign an important role in spasticity to reticulo-spinal facilitation, it is well-known that hyperactivity can come to characterize the reflexes of lower extremities in chronic paraplegia in man. It may be presumed that intrinsically spinal facilitatory mechanisms and, possibly, sensitization of denervation as well, develop in such circumstances and are responsible.

NATURE OF INHIBITION

A century ago, when Sechenov (1863) spent the winter of 1862 in Claude Bernard's laboratory in Paris and, in experiments with the frog, was able to block reflex withdrawal of the leg by stimulating the brain stem, he discovered central neural inhibition and the reticulo-spinal system, as well (Fig. 5, right). Significant insight into the inhibitory process was deferred until 1946, however, when Renshaw (1946) found antidromic inhibition of spinal motoneurons to be associated with interneuronal discharge, evoked by Golgi's recurrent collaterals from the excited motor axons (Fig. 9, left). Shortly thereafter, by applying the method of intracellular microelectrode recording, Eccles and his associates (1957) discovered the neural inhibitory process to be the reciprocal of excitation, i.e., to depend upon hyperpolarization, or increased conductance of the neuronal membrane, preventing a level of depolarization leading to discharge. In Figure 17, a series of intracellular records from a spinal motoneuron, obtained by Coombs, Eccles and Fatt (1955) illustrate hyperpolarization of the post-synaptic membrane in inhibitory synaptic action. In each instance (A-J), the upper trace is a macroelectrode record from the L6 dorsal root, while the lower trace is an intracellular record from a hamstring motoneuron, with upward deflection indicating membrane depolarization. The familiar depolarization of excitation, evoked by an afferent volley from the hamstring muscle, is seen in record J. In record I, an afferent volley from the antagonist quadriceps muscle evokes reciprocal inhibition and a contrasting hyperpolarization of the neuronal membrane is seen. When tested by afferent hamstring stimulation, for an interval of about two milliseconds after hyperpolarization is initiated, the neuron is incapable of being excited (records D to F). Thereafter, excitation is unaffected (rec-

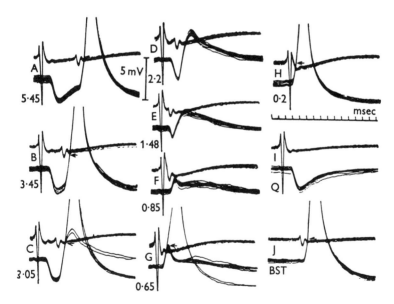

Fig. 17. Oscilloscope records from L6 dorsal root (upper beam) and interior of biceps-semitendinosus neuron in spinal cord of cat (lower beam), showing excitation upon stimulation of afferent nerve from that muscle (J) and inhibition on stimulation of nerve from antagonist quadriceps (I); upward deflection indicating membrane depolarization. Records A-H show interaction of responses to contrasting stimuli presented at the intervals indicated. From Coombs, Eccles and Fatt (1955).

ords A to C) and, when excitation precedes, no interaction occurs (record H).

Eccles and his associates confirmed the related discharge of
interneurons observed by Renshaw during inhibition and went
on to propose their role as chemical commutators, elaborating
an inhibitory transmitter substance responsible for hyperpolarization of the post-synaptic motoneuronal membrane. In the peripheral nervous system, they pointed out, the Dale-Feldberg law
holds that an identical chemical transmitter is liberated at all the
junctional terminals of a single neuron. In Renshaw's experiments on antidromic inhibition, they reasoned, the synaptic transmitter by which the motor axon collateral activated interneurons
must have been identical with that by which its peripheral terminal branches activated muscle, i.e., as the peripheral transmitter was excitatory, so was that from the collateral terminal
to the interneuron. "The interpolation of such an interneuron,"
Eccles and his associates proposed, "can be regarded as a com-
mutator-like device, for changing the chemical transmitter operating on the next cell in the pathway; cells liberating excitatory
transmitter giving place to cells liberating inhibitory transmitter."
In this view, such interneuronal "Renshaw cells" must be present
at the final stage of every neural pathway leading to inhibition.

A diagram, from Eccles, Fatt and Koketsu (1954), summar-
izes the postulated sequence of events from an antidromic impulse in a motor axon to the inhibition of the neuron (Fig. 18).
Shown from above downward are: (a) the action potential in
the motor axon collateral; (b) the concentration of acetylcholine
which it liberates at the axon terminal; (c) the evoked repetitive
firing of the Renshaw cell, superimposed upon background depolarization; (d) the concentration of inhibitory transmitter substance liberated by these impulses at the presynaptic terminals
of the Renshaw cell axon; (e) the hyperpolarization of the motoneuronal membrane induced by this inhibitory transmitter; and
(f) its intensification by bombardment from many Renshaw cells.

These exciting developments in the inhibitory field have stimulated search for the chemical transmitter proposed to be involved. Gamma-aminobutyric acid (GABA) appeared to be a
likely candidate for a time. Its central administration simulated

neural inhibition, while increased excitability and seizure induction followed its depletion. At a recent symposium on GABA and neural inhibition, however, Curtis and Watkins (1960) concluded that GABA depressed neuronal excitability by increasing membrane conductance and shunting of post-synaptic currents, without the induction of hyperpolarization. Additionally, Terzuolo, Sigg and Killam (1960) reported the post-synaptic hyperpolarization of inhibited motoneurons to be unimpaired by thiosemicarbazide-induced depletion of GABA to the point of seizure discharge. From these and other findings, it may be concluded that the specialized inhibitory transmitter substance proposed by recent studies is still to be identified.

RETICULO-SPINAL ACTION

When Eccles (1957) found that the hyperpolarizing inhibitory transmitter substance was antagonized by strychnine, which

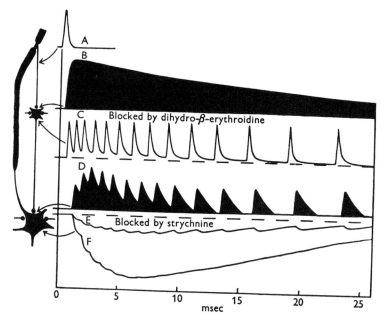

Fig. 18. Diagram summarizing postulated sequence of events from an impulse in a motor axon to the inhibition of a motoneuron (see text). All events are plotted on the same time scale and are referred to histological structures at the left. From Eccles, Fatt and Koketsu (1954).

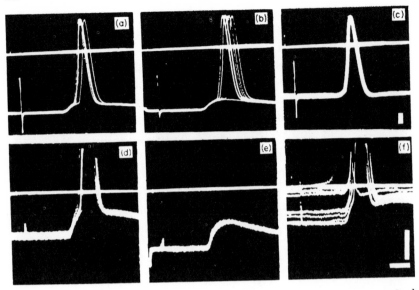

Fig. 19. Intracellular records from a gastrocnemius motor neuron, excited reflexly at 1/sec (sweeps superimposed), before (a— low gain; d— high gain), during (b, e), and after (c, f) stimulation of the anterior lobe of the cerebellum. During threshold cerebellar excitation, the motor neuron discharge is delayed (b); with higher stimulus intensity, there is an increase in membrane potential preventing discharge (e), but no individual hyperpolarizing responses. Time — 1 msec.; calibration — 10 mv. From Terzuolo (1960).

he described as "the curare of the Renshaw cell system," earlier experiments of Terzuolo and Gernandt (1956) showing reticular inhibition of spinal strychnine tetanus suggested that some mechanism other than hyperpolarization of spinal motoneurons was involved. More recently, Terzuolo (1960) has obtained intracellular records from spinal motoneurons during cerebellar inhibition of decerebrate rigidity, probably mediated by the bulbar reticular formation. With increasing intensity of cerebellar stimulation, reflex excitation of discharge was first delayed and then prevented (Fig. 19), but without evocation of individual hyperpolarizing potentials. Koizumi, Ushiyama and Brooks (1959) similarly failed to observe hyperpolarization of the postsynaptic membrane during inhibition of spinal motoneurons induced by reticular stimulation. More recently, Eccles (1961) has proposed a category of pre-synaptic inhibition to account for instances when hyperpolarization of the post-synaptic membrane does not occur.

During contrasting reticular facilitation of spinal reflexes, Renshaw-cell discharge was inhibited, minature potentials of the motor neuron increased in number and fused, and the latency of motoneuron firing was reduced, as though a shift in background excitability had occurred (Koizumi *et al.*, 1959). These findings corroborate the earlier demonstration by Lloyd (1946) that reticulo-spinal facilitation involves processes both of spatial and temporal summation, which proceed directly at the motoneuron itself and to a larger extent through its amplified bombardment by local interneuronal excitation.

GAMMA EFFERENTS AND MUSCLE SPINDLE REGULATION

A second recent development of the greatest interest for an understanding of postural mechanisms has grown from discovery of a gamma-efferent innervation of the intrafusal fibers within the muscle spindle, together with the observation that their tension determines the frequency of afferent firing from this receptor (Granit, 1955). This gamma system, comprising as much as one-third of the ventral root outflow at some spinal levels, forms part of a feedback loop by which the central nervous system can regulate its own proprioceptive input and, in this way, reflexly modify alpha-motor discharge responsible both for the postural and the phasic contraction of muscle (Fig. 20).

With discovery of this mechanism, Granit and Kaada (1952) and Eldred, Granit and Merton (1953) next determined that reticulospinal influences could markedly increase or reduce the firing of the gamma supply to muscle spindles, and so modify input from them. Figure 21, from their publication (1953) shows from left to right: (a) the control rate of firing of a single afferent fiber from a muscle spindle, subjected to four stages of increasing stretch; (b) the great increase of its firing at each stage during background stimulation of the facilitatory reticulospinal system; (c) the great reduction of its firing rate or its failure to fire when gamma discharge is reduced by the inhibitory reticulospinal sys-

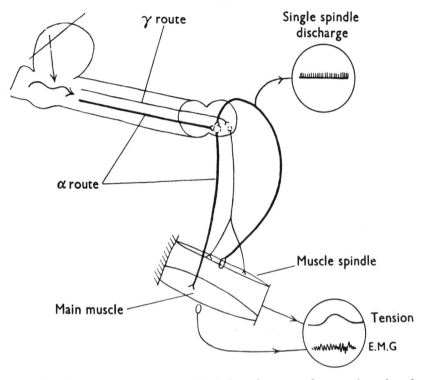

Fig. 20. Diagram of gamma feedback loop between the spinal cord and muscle, together with the cerebellar control of alpha and gamma motor discharge. From Granit, Holmgren and Merton (1955).

tem; and (d) loss or reduction of firing to about the same degree when the spindle was stretched after de-efferentation. It is apparent that this capacity to influence proprioceptive feedback from muscle spindles, by facilitation or inhibition of gamma-motor discharge, provides reticulospinal mechanisms with an additional powerful means of modifying motor performance, over and above effects exerted directly upon alpha motor outflows, or upon spinal interneurons influencing them.

In further analysis, Granit *et al.* (1955) have shown that gamma control from the midbrain tegmentum is effected by two pathways, one fast and one slow. The fast pathway is effective in driving gamma discharge upon single shock stimulation and is proposed to serve the cooperation of gamma and spindle effects

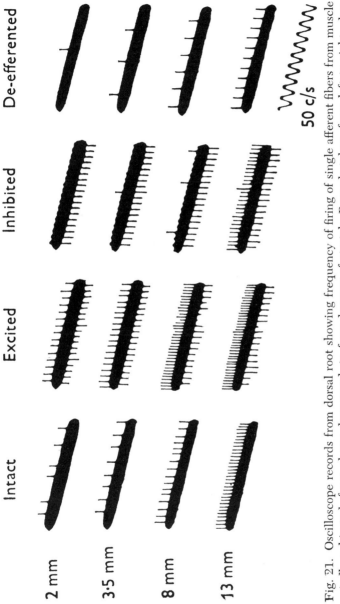

Fig. 21. Oscilloscope records from dorsal root showing frequency of firing of single afferent fibers from muscle spindle subjected, from above downward, to four degrees of stretch. Records taken, from left to right: during control state (intact), during stimulation of facilitatory reticular area (excited), during stimulation of inhibitory reticular area (inhibited), and after section of motor root (deefferented). Facilitation and inhibition of spindle discharge results from reticulospinal influences upon gamma efferent supply to spindle (shock artifact downwards). From Eldred, Granit and Merton (1953).

with rapid movement. The slow path, which requires iterative stimulation of the brain stem and responds in a recruiting fashion, is proposed to serve the volume control of tonic or postural activity. Extension of this program has thrown important light upon decerebrate rigidity and the role of the cerebellum in controlling the linkage between gamma and alpha discharge in postural contraction. Granit, Holmgren and Merton (1955) point out: "It was one of Sherrington's fundamental observations that the state of exaggerated posture he called decerebrate rigidity was dissolved by dorsal root section. This is easily understood if rigidity is due to hyperactivity in the gamma system. . . Pollack and Davis found, however, that in cats decerebrated by the anemic method (so as to render the anterior cerebellum functionless), the rigidity remained after deafferentation. Such rigidity must, therefore, be due mainly to excitation over the alpha route, by-passing the gamma mechanism. . . The rigidity before and the rigidity after cerebellectomy, thus depend upon two essentially different patterns of excitation, the former being predominantly gamma driven, while the latter, which persists after paralysis of the gamma system, is due to primary activity in alpha mechanisms."

From their findings, Granit and his associates (1955) propose that the normal link synchronizing alpha and gamma reflexes is broken by anterior cerebellectomy. The cerebellum, they suggest, controls a neural switch (Fig. 20) which directs excitation either into the alpha or the gamma route. The spindle paralysis produced by experimental cerebellar ablation, in which the muscle is deprived of the services of its length measuring, servo-mechanism, probably accounts for the dysmetria characteristic of cerebellar disease in man.

Because the activity of the gamma efferent system has been found to be related closely to general levels of activity in the CNS (Buchwald and Eldred, 1961) and to provide a substrate for behavioral conditioning (Buchwald, Beatty and Eldred, 1961), it would seem desirable to make greater effort to involve and manipulate the gamma system in muscular training and rehabilitation in physical education and physical therapy in man.

REFERENCES

Allen, W. F.: Formatio reticularis and reticulo-spinal tracts, their visceral functions and possible relationships to tonicity and clonic contractions. *J. Wash. Acad. Sci.*, 22:490-495, 1932.

Buchwald, J. S., Beatty, D. and Eldred, E.: Conditioned responses of gamma and alpha motoneurons in the cat trained to conditioned avoidance. *Exp. Neurol.*, 4:91-105, 1961.

Buchwald, J. S. and Eldred, E.: Relations between gamma efferent discharge and cortical activity. *EEG Clin. Neurophysiol.*, 13:243-247, 1961.

Coombs, J. S., Eccles, J. C. and Fatt, P.: The inhibitory suppression of reflex discharges from motoneurons. *J. Physiol.*, 130:396-413, 1955.

Curtis, D. R. and Watkins, J. C.: Investigations upon the possible synaptic transmitter function of gamma-amino butyric acid and other naturally occurring amino acids. Pp. 424-444. In Roberts, E. (Ed.) *Inhibition in the Nervous System and GABA*. Pergamon, New York, 1960.

Eccles, J. C.: *The Physiology of Nerve Cells*. Johns Hopkins Press, Baltimore, 1957.

Eccles, J. C.: The mechanism of synaptic transmission. *Ergbn. Physiol.*, 51:299-430, 1961.

Eccles, J. C., Fatt, P. and Koketsu, K.: Cholinergic and inhibitory synapses in a pathway from motor-axon collateral to motoneurons. *J. Physiol.*, 126:524-562, 1954.

Eldred, E., Granit, R. and Merton, P. A.: Supraspinal control of the muscle spindles and its significance. *J. Physiol.*, 122:498-523, 1953.

Gernandt, B. E. and Thulin, C. A.: Reciprocal effects upon spinal motoneurons from stimulation of bulbar reticular formation. *J. Neurophysiol.*, 18:113-129, 1955.

Granit, R.: *Receptors and Sensory Perception*. Yale University Press, New Haven, 1955.

Granit, R., Holmgren, B. and Merton, P. A.: The two routes for excitation of muscle and their subservience to the cerebellum. *J. Physiol.*, 130:213-224, 1955.

Granit, R. and Kaada, B. R.: Influence of stimulation of central nervous structures on muscle spindles in cat. *Acta physiol. scandinav.*, 27:130-160, 1952.

Hugelin, A. and Bonvallet, M.: Tonus cortical et contrôle de la facilitation motrice d'origine réticulaire. *J. Physiol. Paris*, 49:1171-1200, 1957.

Koizumi, K., Ushiyama, J. and Brooks, C. M.: A study of reticular formation action on spinal interneurons and motoneurons. *Jap. J. Physiol.*, 9:282-303, 1959.

Lindsley, D. B., Bowden, J. and Magoun, H. W.: Effect upon the EEG of acute injury to the brain stem activating system. *EEG Clin. Neurophysiol.*, 1:475-486, 1949.

Lloyd, D. P. C.: Facilitation and inhibition of spinal motoneurons. *J. Neurophysiol.*, 9:421-438, 1946.

Magoun, H. W.: Caudal and cephalic influences of the brain stem reticular formation. *Physiol. Rev.*, 30:459-474, 1950.

Magoun, H. W. and Rhines, R.: *Spasticity: The Stretch Reflex and Extrapyramidal Systems.* Thomas, Springfield, Illinois, 1948.

Papez, J. W.: Reticulo-spinal tracts in the cat. *J. Comp. Neurol.*, 41:365-399, 1926.

Renshaw, B.: Central effects of centripetal impulses in axons of spinal ventral roots. *J. Neurophysiol.*, 9:191-204, 1946.

Rhines, R. and Magoun, H. W.: Brain stem facilitation of cortical motor response. *J. Neurophysiol.*, 9:219-229, 1946.

Sechenov, I.: *Selected Works.* A. A. Subkov (Ed.) Moscow-Leningrad, 1935.

Sprague, J. M. and Chambers, W. W.: Control of posture by reticular formation and cerebellum in the intact anesthetized and unanesthetized and in the decerebrated cat. *Am. J. Physiol.*, 176:52-64, 1954.

Terzuolo, C. A.: Inhibitory action of the anterior lobe of the cerebellum. Pp. 40-42. In: Roberts, E. (Ed.) *Inhibitions in the Nervous System and GABA.* Pergamon Press, New York, 1960.

Terzuolo, C. A. and Gernandt, B. E.: Spinal unit activity during synchronization of a convulsive type (strychnine tetanus). *Am. J. Physiol.*, 186: 263-270, 1956.

Terzuolo, C. A., Sigg, B. and Killam, K. F.: Effect of thiosemicarbazide on responses of spinal motoneuron. Pp. 336-7. In Roberts, E. (Ed.) *Inhibitions in the Nervous System and GABA.* Pergamon Press, New York, 1960.

3

RETICULO - HYPOTHALAMIC INFLUENCES UPON ENDOCRINE AND VISCERAL FUNCTIONS

At the beginning of the nineteenth century, Bichat (1809) revived interest in the differentiation of an internal or organic life "common both to the vegetable and animal," from an external or animal one "peculiar to the latter alone." Many contributions have since identified the important role of bulbar and hypothalamic mechanisms which regulate visceral functions by way of reticulo-spinal influences upon autonomic as well as somatic motor outflows from the cord.

From more recent study, it is additionally clear that hypothalamic influences exerted by way of the anterior pituitary gland are similarly importantly involved in visceral regulation. Contemporary neuroendocrinologists have rediscovered the ancient *rete mirabile* at the base of the brain, but in the form of portal vessels surrounding the infundibular stalk (Belloni, 1958). This vascular shunt conveys transmitter substances from the hypothalamus to the adenohypophysis where they induce the secretion of tropic hormones. These, in turn, initiate activity at distant target endocrine glands. In current view, hypothalamico-hypophysial relations resemble a kind of protracted neuromuscular junction, in which two linked capillary beds are interposed between pre- and post-synaptic membranes. The first collects transmitter substances from terminals of neurons around the base of the third ventricle, the portal link conveys them to the pituitary, where a second capillary plexus distributes them to receptor sites upon post-synaptic membranes of adenohypophysial cells.

The characteristically differential secretion of each of the several pituitary hormones implies some biochemical specificity, either of transmitter substance or of receptor site. Both the indi-

vidualized responses to different afferent stimuli and the spatial
representation of hypothalamic areas involved suggest that considerable differentiation has already been established on the
neural side. Cold stimuli, for example, can evoke the secretion
of thyrotropic hormone and stressful stimuli that of adreno-
corticotropic hormone, in each case without secretion of gonado-
tropic hormone and indeed with its reciprocal inhibition. Just
as alpha, gamma and preganglionic autonomic motoneurons, in-
nervating different categories of effectors, occupy distinct areas
of the spinal gray matter, so a kind of glandulotopic distribution
of function can be recognized in the neural aggregates forming
the floor of the third ventricle. Regions concerned with TSH,
ACTH and FSH are located from before backwards through the
hypothalamus; consideration can be given to each of them in
turn, beginning with regulation of secretion of the adrenocortico-
tropic hormone, ACTH.

REGULATION OF PITUITARY-ADRENOCORTICAL ACTIVITY

Interest in pituitary-adrenocortical involvement in "stress"
(Selye, 1950), as well as in adrenal replacement therapy in disease, has stimulated study of hypothalamic control of the secretion of ACTH by the pituitary. As seen in Figure 22 from Sayers
(1957), ACTH is elaborated both in response to a variety of
"stressful" stimuli, conveyed to the hypothalamus through the
central core of the brain stem (Anderson, Haymaker *et al.*, 1957)
and, additionally, as a consequence of "psychological stress," in
which corticifugal or limbic projections to the cephalic brain stem
are probably involved. Furthermore, ACTH release can be induced by circulating epinephrine, with which is associated a
pronounced increase in resting activity in the posterior hypothalamus (Porter, 1953). Direct electrical stimulation of this
same neural region evokes secretion of ACTH and, following
injury to tuberal and posterior hypothalamic areas, stressful
stimulation is no longer productive of ACTH secretion (Porter,
1954).

The nature of the transmitter substance responsible for the
secretion of corticotropin from the adenohypophysis is still un-

known. Slusher and Roberts (1954) have prepared effective lip-ide or lipoprotein fractions from the posterior hypothalamus. Others have presented evidence for a peptide, like those of the posterior pituitary, as the specific corticotropin releasing factor. Both the vasopressor and antidiuretic hormones of the neuro-hypophysis have also been proposed to be involved in the secre-tion of ACTH (Ganong, 1959).

GASTROINTESTINAL AND CARDIOVASCULAR PATHOLOGY

The studies of French, Porter and their associates (1953) have revealed dual routes by which hypothalamic influences can increase gastric hydrochloric acid secretion. In the waking monkey, focal stimulation of the anterior hypothalamus yielded a vagus mediated HCl secretion, peaking in one hour; while pos-

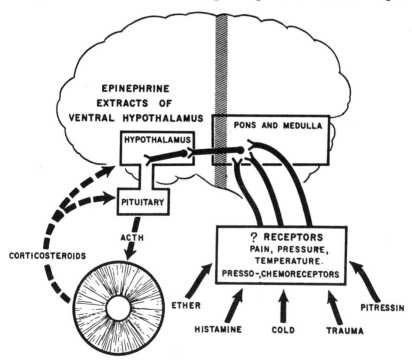

Fig. 22. Schematized representation of the neuroendocrine relations in-volved in the control of pituitary-adrenocortical activity. From Sayers (1957).

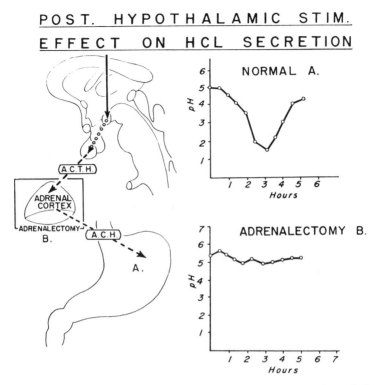

Fig. 23. Diagram (*left*) showing route by which posterior hypothalamic stimulation can induce secretion of gastric HCl. Graph (*right*) showing secretion of gastric HCl (fall in pH), reaching peak three hours after hypothalamic stimulation (A), and the block of secretion by adrenalectomy (B). From French, Longmire, Porter and Movius (1953).

terior hypothalamic stimulation yielded HCl secretion peaking in three hours, mediated by the pituitary and adrenal cortex (Fig. 23). This latter closely resembled the rise in gastric hydrochloric acid secretion induced by the direct administration of ACTH or ACH. Insulin hypoglycemia was found to augment gastric HCl by both routes and its dual effects could be differentiated respectively by vagotomy or adrenalectomy.

The commonly held view that prolonged and excessive secretion of gastric hydrochloric acid is the causal factor in gastroduodenal ulcer led French, Porter and their associates (1954) to implant electrodes in the monkey's hypothalamus and to stimulate this region at four-hour intervals around the clock for periods of one to three months. In the initial series of ten animals, six showed signs of gastrointestinal pathology and, in four of these, frank ulcers were found in the pyloric stomach or first segment of the duodenum (Fig. 24). It was concluded that while the hypothalamic-pituitary mechanism involved in provoking increase in ACTH and ACH secretion may normally be of benefit in response to stress, its chronically maintained excitation may be responsible for the production of one type of so-called psychosomatic disease, gastric ulcer.

This work was extended by Porter and associates (1958) to a study of the effects of psychological stress. In chronic conditioning experiments, two monkeys were yoked in adjacent chairs so that one was responsible for undertaking all avoidance procedures for the pair. During alternating six-hour sessions

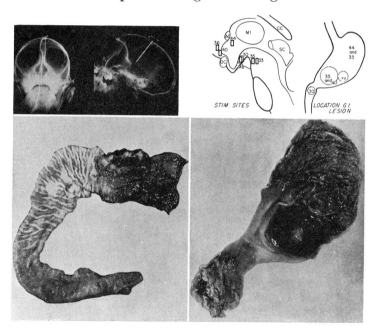

Fig. 24. Ulceration of duodenum (*lower left*) and pylorus (*lower right*) induced in monkeys by prolonged hypothalamic stimulation through implanted electrodes (*upper left*). The sites of hypothalamic stimulation and distribution of gastrointestinal pathology in six animals are shown in **upper right**. From French, Porter, Cavanaugh and Longmire (1954).

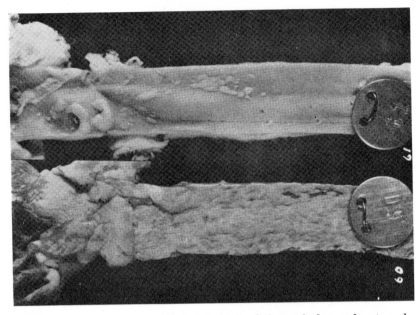

Fig. 25. Aortas of two rabbits fed high cholesterol diets, showing the marked atherosclerotic effect of additional chronic stimulation of the hypothalamus (*below*). From Gunn, Friedman and Byers (1960).

around the clock, this "executive" monkey had to push a lever to avoid a recurring shock, both to its own and to its associate's feet. Although the executive animals maintained rates of lever-pressing considerably higher than necessary and so avoided all but an occasional shock, the psychological toll was great. While the passive members of the pairs showed no abnormality, two of the executive animals developed duodenal ulcers after three weeks, leading, in one, to a fatal perforation.

Comparable experimentation has begun to explore neurogenic factors involved in atherosclerosis and hypertension. The work of Gunn, Friedman and Byers (1960) has shown that in a group of rabbits fed a cholesterol-rich diet, those with daily stimulation of the tuberal hypothalamus over a period of three months consistently displayed higher serum lipid levels and, terminally, exhibited a strikingly more severe aortic atherosclerosis than did the unstimulated controls (Fig. 25). In the survey of neurophysiological factors in hypertension, Anokhin (1960) has discussed factors which determine the level of excitability of central vasomotor mechanisms as follows: "In the vasomotor center, there is a clash of two inflows, one from above which is the final result of the activity of billions of cortical and subcortical cells; the other from many peripheral vascular baroreceptors with, however, a limited maximal impulse-firing rate. We can consider the process as two pans of a balance. Under normal conditions of life, depressor impulses always overbalance and the vasoconstrictor center is inhibited. The entire process of development of an hypertensive state, in relation to the formation of dominant and permanent excitation at a cortico-subcortical level, would mean an overbalance of the central side of the scale, which cannot be counteracted by depressor impulses from the periphery."

REGULATION OF PITUITARY-THYROID ACTIVITY

While the pituitary appears to have a relatively greater degree of autonomous function with respect to thyrotropin (TSH) than with the secretion of other tropic hormones, electrical stimulation of the hypothalamus can accelerate thyroxine production in the rabbit and cat (Fig. 26; Bogdanove, 1962). Hypothalamic lesions block the increased elaboration of TSH and thyroxine induced by exposure to cold (Knigge, 1960) and such hypothalamic injury also prevents the thyroid response to goitrogens. Although the TSH-regulating mechanism may be rather diffusely represented, the anterior hypothalamus seems the region most involved.

An inhibition of thyrotropin secretion, induced by local injection of adrenalin into the mammillary body (von Euler and Holmgren, 1956) was not affected by reserpine, nor was it reproduced by norepinephrine or dopamine (Harrison, 1961). This may be related to the stimulating action of adrenalin on ACTH secretion, mediated by the posterior hypothalamus, and the reciprocally inhibitory relations that seem to exist between the hypothalamic mechanisms influencing the secretion of different pituitary hormones. Such neural inhibition is evidently not implicated in the negative feedback by which rising titers of circulating thyroxine reduce TSH secretion, for the injection studies

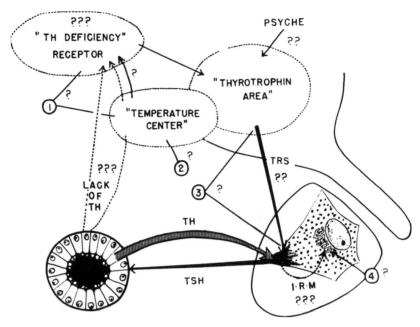

Fig. 26. Schematized representation of the neuroendocrine relations involved in the control of pituitary-thyroid activity. From Bogdanove (1962).

of von Euler and Holmgren (1956) and Harrison (1961) indicate that this is managed directly at the pituitary level.

REGULATION OF PITUITARY-GONADAL ACTIVITY

The recent work of Sawyer and his associates (1957, 1959, 1961) has greatly clarified the chain of events by which the brain evokes the surge of gonadotropin from the pituitary which leads to ovulation. In the estrous cat or rabbit, in which this mechanism is normally triggererd by coitus, vaginal stimulation is followed by a marked and prolonged alteration in the electrical activity of the basal forebrain and anterior hypothalamus. In the intrinsically recurring reproductive cycle of the rat, similar changes in electrical activity are seen at a fixed time of the day preceding ovulation. Spontaneous or hormonally induced estrous is necessary for this display, which is presumed to initiate the release of pituitary gonadotropin and so trigger ovulation. In all forms, the final common pathway for this gonadotropin-releasing ovulatory influence involves tuberal structures located just above the median eminence of the stalk. In both the rabbit and cat, ovulation can be induced by stimulating this region and experimental lesions here block ovulation following coitus (Fig. 27). In the rat, the gonadotropin-releasing mechanism may additionally extend backward to involve the midbrain and the region of the mammillary peduncle as well (Critchlow, 1958).

Sawyer and his associates (1961) have accumulated a large body of pharmacological information relating to hypothalamic-gonadal function. In both the rat and rabbit, ovulation can be prevented by the appropriately timed administration of atropine, pentobarbital, morphine and chlorpromazine. The doses employed induced a sleep-like EEG, as well as an elevation of arousal threshold, and their prevention of ovulation was earlier attributed to impairment of conduction of ascending reticular impulses responsible for activating the pituitary stimulating mechanism. More recently, Sawyer (1961) has found, however, that the induction of ovulation by direct electrical stimulation of the hypothalamus, at the last neural step before the portal system, can also be prevented by these substances which, it should be noted, include the cholinergic blocking agent, atropine. The adrenergic blocking agents SKF-501 and reserpine, which are effective in preventing ovulation in the normal animal, do not block the ovulatory effect of such direct hypothalamic stimulation. These recent findings imply that the hypothalamic-gonadotropin releasing substance is a cholinergic one. They suggest also that the adrenergic link normally present in the afferent induction of ovulation is somewhere proximal to the cholinergic one, rather than distal to it as previously proposed.

Recent observations of Davidson and Sawyer (1961) have determined the self-regulatory process by which rising titers of circulating gonadal hormones check the further secretion of pituitary gonadotropins. The hypothalamus is importantly implicated in this succession of events, for implantation of crystals of estrogen in the median eminence and tuberal region of female rabbits inhibited copulation-induced ovulation and led to ovarian atrophy (Fig. 28). Such animals nevertheless continued to accept the male eagerly and displayed an unusual degree of

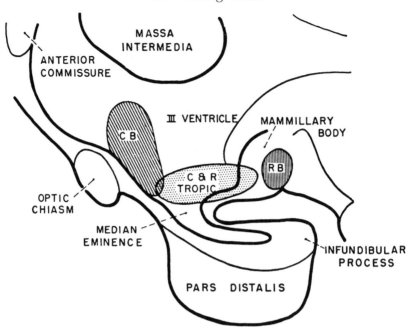

Fig. 27. Midsagittal view of hypothalamus and pituitary showing the common tuberal area controlling release of pituitary ovulating hormone in both the cat and rabbit (C & R, TROPIC); and the areas concerned with sexual behavior, in the anterior hypothalamus of the cat (CB) and the posterior hypothalamus of the rabbit (RB). From Sawyer and Kawakami (1961).

frequency of sexual behavior. In the dog, analogous findings were obtained in the male, in which implantation of testosterone into the same tuberal hypothalamic region resulted in aspermia and pronounced testicular and prostatic atrophy. Implantation into other neural sites, or into the pituitary itself, failed to produce these results. The experiments support the view that, in the manner of a negative feedback, circulating gonadal hormones normally act back upon the tuberal portion of the hypothalamus to check the further secretion of gonadotropins.

Such "pharmacological" influences of circulating endocrine hormones which, in the manner of automatic control theory, have come to employ inverse feedback to regulate performance, are currently being applied to the development of an effective oral

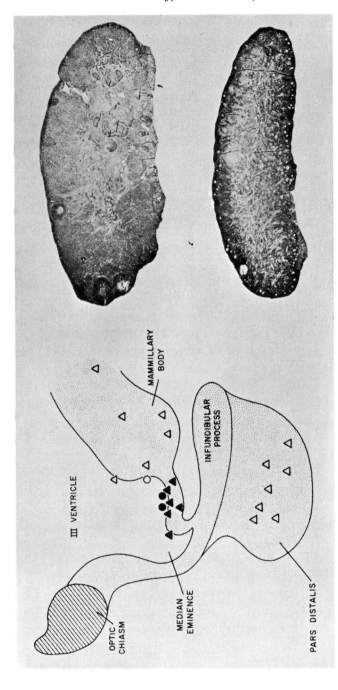

Fig. 28. Midsagittal view of rabbit's hypothalamus and pituitary (*left*), with black symbols marking the location of estrogen implants which blocked copulation-induced ovulation and eventually led to ovarian atrophy (*right, below*), by comparison with the normal control (*right, above*). From Davidson and Sawyer (1961).

contraceptive in man, or rather, in woman. The new progestational antifertility agents, including norethynodrel and norethisterone, which have proven effective in preventing conception in women, have been found to elevate the threshold of the hypothalamic gonadotropin releasing mechanism in the rabbit and to block ovulation by this means. Their antifertility properties thus appear referable to effects upon the brain, rather than to to direct modification of ovarian function as was earlier conceived.

As contraceptives, these antifertility agents take advantage of the existence of the dual and functionally distinct hypothalamic mechanisms for sexual activity, so as to block the tuberal system serving the induction of ovulation, while leaving unaffected the spatially separate mechanisms serving the consummatory stages of mating behavior (Fig. 27). In addition, brain mechanisms serving libido and the appetitive aspects of sexual activity are similarly uninvolved, so that both the inclination for mating and its behavioral performance are unaffected, while consequent gonadotropin-release and ovulation fail to occur. Fertility depends upon the sequential stages by which sexual excitement and mating normally induce gonadotropin release and consequent ovulation. The antifertility agents are effective by virtue of failing to act upon the initial behavioral phase of the sequence, while they block the succeeding endocrine phase, at the stage of elaboration of the gonadotropin-releasing factor from the hypothalamus.

In this respect, the action of these antifertility agents closely resembles that of the progestational steroids normally elaborated by the ovary during gestation which, conveyed by the systemic circulation to the brain, prevent ovulation throughout the period of pregnancy. There is a paradoxical element in the circumstance that, by pharmacological means, the human female is now able to simulate an aspect of pregnancy, in order to prevent conception.

REFERENCES

Anderson, E., Bates, R. W., Hawthorne, E., Haymaker, W., Knowlton, K., Rioch, D. Mck., Spence, W. T. and Wilson, H.: The effect of midbrain and spinal cord transection on endocrine and metabolic functions, with postulation of a midbrain hypothalamico-pituitary activating system. *Recent Progresss in Hormone Research, 13:*21-66, 1957.

Anokhin, P. K.: The physiological basis or the pathogenesis of hypertensive states. *Cor et Vasa,* 2:247-272, 1960.

Belloni, L.: *Rete mirabile* (introduzione Storica). In *Pathophysiologia Diensephalica,* pp. 1-17. Springer-Velny, Wien, 1958.

Bichat, X.: *Physiological Researches upon Life and Death.* Watkins, T. (Tr.) Smith and Maxwell, Philadelphia, 1809.

Bogdanove, E. M.: Regulation of TSH secretion. *Fed. Proc., 21:*623-627, 1962.

Critchlow, V.: Blockade of ovulation in the rat by mesencephalic lesions. *Endocrinology, 63:*596-610, 1958.

Davidson, J. M. and Sawyer, C. H.: Effects of localized intracerebral implantation of estrogen on reproductive function in the female rabbit. *Acta endocrinol.,* 37:385-393, 1961.

Euler, C. von and Holmgren, B.: The role of hypothalamo-hypophysial connexions in thyroid secretion. *J. Physiol., 131:*137-146, 1956.

French, J. D., Longmire, R. L., Porter, R. W. and Movius, H. J.: Extra-vagal influences and gastric hydrochloric acid secretion induced by stress stimuli. *Surgery,* 34:621-632, 1953.

French, J. D., Porter, R. W., Cavanaugh, E. B. and Longmire, R. L.: Experimental observations on "psychosomatic" mechanisms. I. Gastro-intestinal disturbances. *Arch. Neurol. & Psychiat. (Chicago),* 72:267-281, 1954.

Ganong, W. F.: Adrenal-hypophyseal interrelations, pp. 187-201, In: Gorham, A. (Ed.) *Comparative Endocrinology,* John Wiley, New York, 1959.

Gunn, C. G., Friedman, M. and Byers, S. O.: Effect of chronic hypo-thalamic stimulation upon cholesterol-induced atteroschlerosis in the rabbit. *J. Clin. Invest., 39:*1963-1972, 1960.

Harrison, T. S.: Some factors influencing thyrotropin release in the rabbit. *Endocrin., 68:*466-478, 1961.

Knigge, K. M.: Neuroendocrine mechanisms influencing ACTH and TSH secretion and their role in cold acclimation. *Fed. Proc., 19:*45-51, 1960.

Porter, R. W.: Hypothalamic involvement in the pituitary-adrenocortical response to stress stimuli. *Am. J. Physiol., 172:*515-519, 1953.

Porter, R. W.: The central nervous system and stress-induced eosinopenia. *Recent Progress in Hormone Research, 10:*1-27, 1954.

Porter, R. W., Brady, J. V., Conrad, D., Mason, J. W., Galambos, R. and Rioch, D. M.: Some experimental observations on gastro-intestinal lesions in behaviorally conditioned monkeys. *Psychosom. Med.,* 20: 379-394, 1958.

Sayers, G.: Factors influencing the level of ACTH in the blood. Pp. 138-149. In: *Ciba Foundation Colloquia on Endocrinology,* vol. II, *Hormones in the Blood,* J. & A. Churchill, London, 1957.

Sawyer, C. H.: Triggering of the pituitary by the C.N.S. Pp. 164-174. In: Bullock, T. H. (Ed.) *Physiological Triggers.* Am. Physiol. Soc., Washington, 1957.

Sawyer, C. H.: Nervous control of ovulation. Pp. 1-20. In: Lloyd, C. W. (Ed.) *Recent Progress in the Endocrinology of Reproduction.* Academic Press, New York, 1959.

Sawyer, C. H. and Kawakami, M.: Interactions between the central nervous system and hormones influencing ovulation. Pp. 79-97. In: Villee, C. A. (Ed.). *Control of Ovulation,* Pergamon Press, New York, 1961.

Selye, H.: *The Physiology and Pathology of Exposure to Stress.* Montreal, 1950.

Slusher, M. A. and Roberts, S.: Fractionation of hypothalamic tissues for pituitary-stimulating activity. *Endocrinol., 55:*245-254, 1954.

4

LIMBIC SYSTEMS FOR INNATE AND EMOTIONAL BEHAVIOR

THERE IS BOTH OLD AND RECENT indication that hypothalamic mechanisms for neuroendocrine and visceral control, together with basal and medial forebrain systems lying immediately upstream of them, are concerned with the management of innate and emotional behavior. Two ideological lines have contributed importantly to current formulations of this view.

The broad biological background was provided by Darwin (1871) who proposed a view of evolution in which each living form adapted to its environment by staking out a territory, in which it obtained food and shelter and so preserved its individual life, and sought a mate and reproduced and reared its young and so preserved its race. For survival of the fittest in this struggle for life, each form additionally found it necessary to combat enemies or predators and, when overpowered, to preserve itself by flight. It was in relation to these basic biological activities, Darwin proposed, that the brain came to contain mechanisms for the management of what MacLean (1958) has more recently called the four "F's": feeding, fighting, fleeing, and undertaking mating activity.

A second line of development was begun by Claude Bernard (1859), when he called attention to the preservation of stability of the internal environment, as a condition of all higher and freer life. The general principle of homeostasis was later proposed by Cannon (1939) in explanation of this internal stability and, with Weiner's (1948) formulation of automatic control theory, it became possible to seek analogies between the physiological processes serving homeostasis and those of a mechanical homeostat. The latter's component parts include a sensor, a central mechanism, possessing a gain-setting bias, and an effector. These

[53]

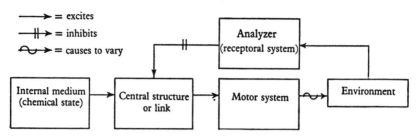

Fig. 29. Diagram of feedback organization by which the constancy of the internal environment is preserved in homeostasis. From Deutsch (1960).

parts are so arranged that alterations induced by the effector feed back to regulate continued performance, either through the sensor or by changing the bias on the central mechanism, or both. Specific applications of this analogy to models of innate behavior (Fig. 29) have recently been provided by Deutsch (1960), Pribram (1961) and Brobeck (1962).

The life and race-preserving pursuits of innate behavior relate closely to the basic appetites and drives, as well as to emotion. Their obtrusive presence throughout the animal series implies management at neural levels established early in phylogeny. Considerable evidence implicates structures called limbic, for their distribution around the attachment of the cerebral hemispheres to the cephalic end of the brain stem. This limbic lobe was identified by Broca (1878), but was first designated as a circuit for emotion by Papez (1937). A succeeding series of contributions by the Yale School (Kaada, 1951; MacLean, 1949; Pribram and Kruger, 1954; Fulton, 1953) have contributed importantly to current views.

INNATE BEHAVIOR

As Kubie (1948) has pointed out, activity related both to feeding and to reproduction has a "biochemical core" and is primarily concerned with "the translation of bodily needs into behavior." These needs are conspicuously cyclic and their periodicity is a feature characteristic of innate behavior. When the activity of the rat is recorded (Richter, 1927), a three-hour cycle can be observed in relation to food intake and a four-day cycle, with a doubling of running activity, to recurring estrous periods (Fig. 30).

Sequential steps have been differentiated within each such behavioral cycle (Tinbergen, 1951). An initial appetitive or exploratory stage is marked by plasticity, adaptiveness and complex integration. In many species, exploration for food or a sexual partner often involves prolonged motor expenditures and, on the perceptual side, enhanced alertness and responsiveness to stimulation. By contrast, the consummatory act itself is usually brief and stereotyped. Following it, satiety typically involves "a state of rest, of disinterest in the outside world, and even of sleep which is in marked contrast to the heightened activity of the appetitive phase" (Dell, 1958). While the exploratory stages of innate behavior must implicate all major components of the brain, integrative mechanisms for the consummatory act and for satiety are more focal. Those for consummation may be considered now, while those for satiety will in large part be deferred to page 162.

ALIMENTARY BEHAVIOR

A remarkably active program of recent experimentation is exploring the limbic and hypothalamic management of alimentary behavior (Anand, 1961). Feeding can be induced by direct electrical stimulation of the lateral hypothalamus (Fig. 31), even in the satiated animal (Larsson, 1954; Andersson, Jewell and Larson, 1958). Aphagia follows lesions here and the lateral portions of the hypothalamus (Anand and Brobeck, 1951), or connections to this region from the globus pallidus (Morgane, 1961), are importantly involved in feeding. Reciprocally, the ventromedial hypothalamic nucleus or region is implicated in satiety. Its direct stimulation stops feeding behavior, even in the hungry animal; while lesions in it are followed by hyperphagia, leading to pronounced obesity (Fig. 32; Hetherington and Ranson, 1940). A negative feedback appears operant in alimentary behavior, by which peripheral stores relay information concerning their inventory to hypothalamic regulatory mechanisms. After lesions were made in the hypothalamic ventromedial nucleus, with resultant hyperphagia and obesity, in one of a pair of para-

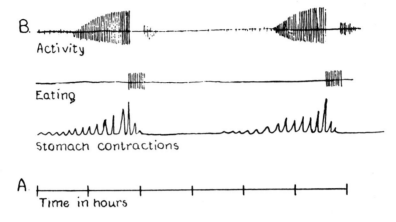

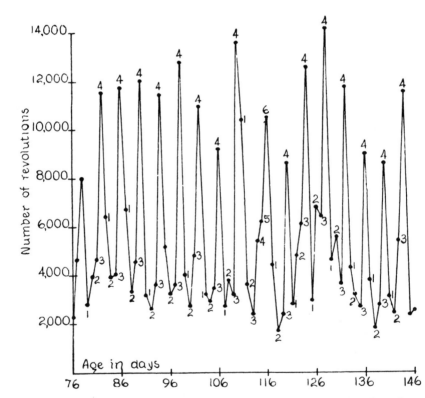

Fig. 30. Records of running activity of the rat, showing the three hour cycle related to food intake (*above*) and the four day cycle related to recurring estrous periods (*below*). From Richter (1927).

biotic rats, the other responded to its mate's overfeeding by eating less and becoming thin (Hervey, 1959).

Food intake tends generally to be correlated with drinking and, while hypothalamic mechanisms for the two are adjacent, they appear to act separately and indeed to depend respectively upon contrasting adrenergic and cholinergic excitation (Grossman, 1960). Andersson and McCann (1955) have identified a region near the paraventricular nucleus of the goat where electrical stimulation, or the injection of hypertonic solutions, evokes a Gargantuan polydipsia, in which as much as sixteen liters of water may be drunk in a single experiment (Fig. 31).

The increased firing of single supraoptic neurons has been observed on intracarotid injection of hypertonic sodium chloride or glucose (Cross and Green, 1959). In addition to these osmotic and glucostatic factors, however, such a variety of other means of influencing these mechanisms has been proposed—by shifts in

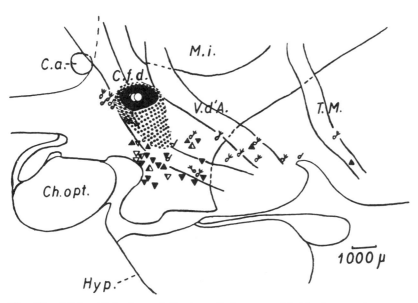

Fig. 31. Midsagittal view of the hypothalamus, with black triangles marking the sites where electrical stimulation caused feeding and the solid black area, drinking, in the goat. Microinjection of hypertonic NaCl, in the dotted area, also caused polydipsia. From Andersson, Jewell and Larsson (1958) and Andersson and McCann (1955).

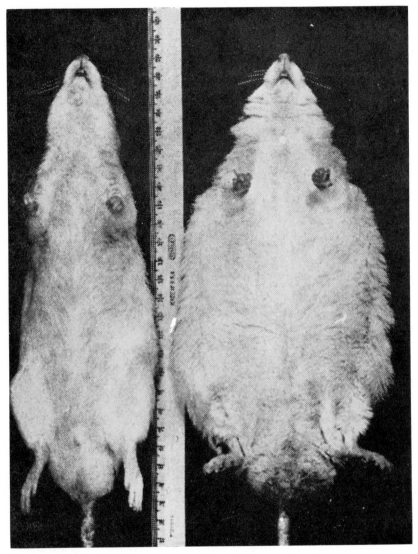

Fig. 32. Photos showing obesity in the rat following lesions in the hypothalamic ventromedial nucleus (*right*), by comparison with the litter mate
control (*left*). From Hetherington & Ranson (1940).

serum lipids or amino acids, by changes in temperature, as well as by afferent stimuli from the oropharynx or digestive tract— that a multiple factor theory for regulating feeding and drinking seems presently most acceptable (Brobeck, 1955).

MATING BEHAVIOR

Turning from food to sex, the hypothalamic management of consummatory patterns of mating behavior are similarly becoming well established from recent work (Sawyer and Kawakami, 1961). As noted earlier, hypothalamic mechanisms integrating mating performance are separate from those regulating pituitary gonadotrophic functions and, in the cat and rabbit, lie in front of and behind them, respectively (Fig. 27). In the female, lesions here are followed by permanent loss of estrus behavior, impossible to overcome by estrogens, although the hypothalamic-pituitary system remains viable and ovarian atrophy does not occur. The enhanced alertness and augmented motor performance during the appetitive or exploratory stage of sexual behavior is associated with an increased excitability of the reticular system. For three to four hours after administration of progesterone (Fig. 33), the EEG arousal threshold was markedly lowered, with a succeeding elevation above the control level. This increased responsiveness was associated with estrus and mating behavior, while the secondary elevation of threshold was correlated with anestrus and absence of sexual responsiveness. This striking modification of neural function, together with that after implanting sex hormones (Harris, Michael and Scott, 1958), suggests that the induction of sexual behavior, together with management of its remarkable periodicity in the estrus cycle, may in large part be accountable in terms of direct endocrine modification of excitability of the brain.

POSITIVE AND NEGATIVE REINFORCEMENT

The impelling nature of innate behavior is explicable also in terms of its built-in drive or motivational content; referable, in turn, to mechanisms for reinforcement, recently discovered in the limbic forebrain and cephalic brain stem. Much had been learned of factors which modify behavior through use of the

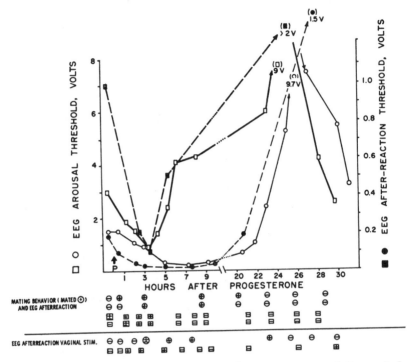

Fig. 33. Graph showing the marked initial increase in excitability and the subsequent pronounced elevation of threshold of the reticular formation and hypothalamus, following injection of progesterone (P) in the rabbit. From Sawyer and Kawakami (1961).

Skinner box, in which an animal pushes a lever to obtain a reward, such as a pellet of food or a drop of milk. Closure with neurophysiology occurred when Olds and Milner (1954) arranged a Skinner box so that, by pushing a lever, an animal with chronically implanted electrodes could deliver a stimulus directly to a part of its own brain (Fig. 34). This inspired innovation revealed the existence of a previously unsuspected, positively-reinforcing mechanism in the basal forebrain, excitation of which appeared to have all the features of primary reward. With appropriate electrode placements, the animal repeatedly stimulated its own brain to the exclusion of all other activity for long periods of time (Olds, 1958). Stimulation rates reaching the astronomical figure of 8,000 self-stimuli per hour occurred with electrodes in the posterior hypothalamus and midbrain; while lower rates of self-stimulation were characteristic of more rostral sites (Fig. 35). Pharmacological distinction was also possible, for tranquilizing agents, such as reserpine or chlorpromazine, reduced or abolished self-stimulation of the posterior hypothalamus, but not of more cephalic structures.

Olds' (1958) animals ran a maze as fast, and a runway faster, for self-stimulation than for food reward. When tested by cross-

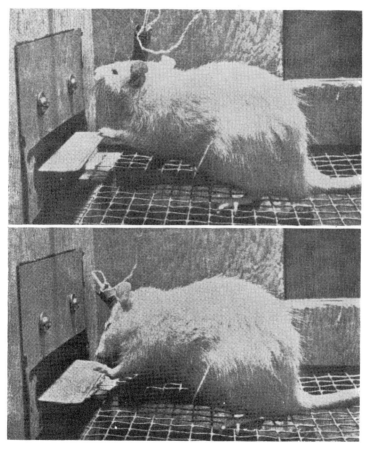

Fig. 34. Rat with electrodes implanted in brain, and with foot upon bar (*above*), presses bar (*below*) and delivers stimulus to its own brain. Animal must release lever and press again to repeat stimulus. Some animals have stimulated themselves for twenty-four hours without rest and as often as 8,000 times an hour. From Olds (1958).

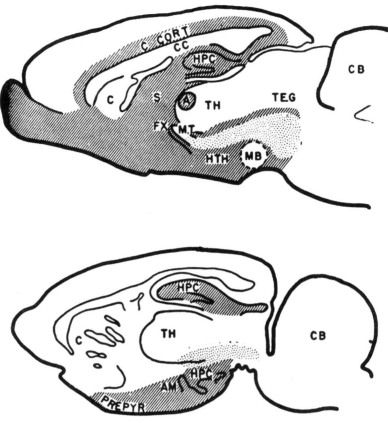

Fig. 35. Parasagittal sections through the brain of the rat showing the distribution of areas for positive (*cross-lined*) and negative (*stippled*) re-inforcement. From Olds (1958).

ing a painful grid, the drive for self-stimulation was at least twice that of a twenty-four-hour hunger drive. Some differentiation of hunger- and sex-reward systems was possible, for rates of self-stimulation of the medial hypothalamus were influenced by hunger or its satiety, while administration of sex hormones or castration modified the rates of self-stimulation of more lateral hypothalamic regions.

With electrodes in an adjacent but more dorsal diencephalic zone, Olds (1958) observed negative reinforcement, in the sense that after an animal had once stimulated this region, it would never do so again (Figs. 35, 37). When this area was repeatedly excited in a characteristic laboratory setting, anticipatory unrest was soon provoked by the setting alone. When trained to do so, an animal would repeatedly turn a wheel or press a lever to avoid stimulation of this part of its brain (Delgado, Roberts and Miller, 1954; Lilly, 1958). When this region was stimulated in a social setting, a cat would vigorously attack its neighbor, suggesting a functional relationship with central mechanisms for aggression.

The conceptual implications of these findings are of the greatest interest. May we presume that these dual, reciprocally antagonistic half-centers for positive and negative reinforcement serve subjective pleasure and pain and their elaborations as reward and punishment? Are slight feelings of pleasure or unpleasantness associated with liminal activity in these systems, while more exquisite or orgiastic enjoyments on the one hand, or intensities of rage and terror on the other, are related to their full-blown excitation? In these studies, have Heaven and Hell been located in the animal brain?

As Olds (1958) has pointed out: "In classical theory, reward has been interpreted as being the falling phase of the same stimulation which at high levels constitutes punishment. Drive and punishment are synonymous, according to this theory, and a reward is held to be fundamentally nothing more than the reduction of a drive. The hedonistic view that behavior is pulled forward by pleasure, as well as pushed forward by pain, is rejected in classical theory for the more parsimonious notion that pain supplies the push and that learning based on pain reduction supplies the direction. . . (Present work) clearly shows one implication of the drive-reduction theory to be incorrect, for massive input to certain parts of the central nervous system can be shown to have rewarding effects. Further, by showing that there are anatomically separate mechanisms for reward and punishment in the brain, it points directly to a physiological basis for the motivational dualism suggested in the hedonistic theory."

AGGRESSIVE BEHAVIOR

Much earlier evidence points to the hypothalamic integra-

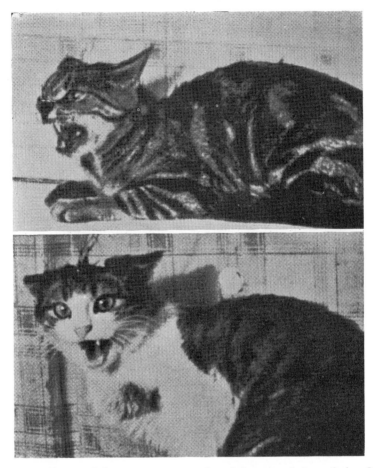

Fig. 36. Affective-defensive reaction induced by stimulation of the diencephalon through implanted electrodes. From Hess (1954).

tion of patterns of aggressive behavior. Coordinate and directed
"affective-defensive responses" (Fig. 36) are readily induced by
lateral hypothalamic stimulation in the intact animal (Hess,
1954; Masserman, 1943; Hunsperger, 1956). In the surviving
decorticate cat, vigorous patterns of sham or quasi-rage may
often be evoked by trivial afferent stimulation (Bard and Rioch,
1937), while such activity is only fragmentary after lower de-
cerebration (Bard and Macht, 1958). In a docile cat, focal lesions of the hypothalamic ventromedial nucleus are followed

by an exaggeration of aggressive tendencies to the point of savagery (Wheatley, 1944). In aggression, as in feeding, the lateral hypothalamus thus appears to be excitatory (Fig. 37) and the medial, inhibitory of behavior.

AMYGDALA

At about the same time that Papez (1937) proposed a limbic circuit for emotion, Klüver and Bucy's (1939) observations of the consequences of bilateral temporal lobectomy initiated current study of this part of the brain. Among the striking alterations

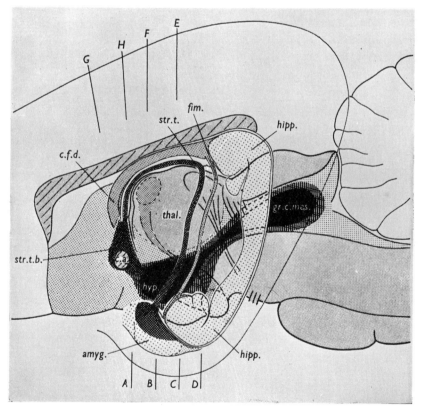

Fig. 37. Reconstruction of the relations of the amygdala and hippocampus to the cephalic brain stem of the cat, with black shading indicating the amygdala, hypothalamic and periaqueductal regions from which affective-defensive responses can be evoked. From Fernandez de Molina and Hunsperger (1959).

in their monkeys, tameness, docility and emotional unresponsiveness were related to a reduction or loss of fear and anger, while hypersexuality and hyperphagia marked exaggeration of these latter categories of behavior. These changes now seem referable to ablation of the amygdala and/or the adjacent pyriform lobe.

In intact animals, stimulation of the amygdala induces fear and rage responses (Kaada, Andersson and Jansen, 1954; Ursin and Kaada, 1960), components of which can be evoked along the course of its efferent stria terminalis to the hypothalamus and midbrain (Fig. 37; Fernandez de Molina and Hunsperger, 1959, 1962). When the two regions are excited concomitantly, the amygdala may suppress attack behavior elicited by hypothalamic stimulation (Egger and Flynn, 1962). Focal lesions of the amygdala or pyriform cortex are followed by docility and hypersexuality in a variety of animals (Schreiner and Kling, 1953). In the cat, however, exaggeration of sexual behavior appeared to consist largely of the display of a normally wide-ranging repertoire outside of the usual territorial limits (Green, Clemente and de Groot, 1957). From a social point of view, amygdala lesions in the monkey are followed by change from a dominant to a submissive position in the group hierarchy (Rosvold, Mirsky and Pribram, 1954).

The amygdala thus appears to serve importantly in regulating the excitability of lower mechanisms for the consummatory phases of innate behavior. If these latter are conceived as homeostats, the amygdala can be proposed to set the bias on their central mechanisms, so as to raise or lower their excitability. The tameness of wild animals and the general loss of aggression following amygdalectomy, suggests that it or the adjacent pyriform cortex exerts a facilitatory influence on lower mechanisms for aggressive behavior. Conversely, the hyperphagia and the hypersexuality, following amygdalectomy, suggests that it exerts a checking or inhibiting influence upon lower mechanisms for alimentary and sexual behavior. Additionally, animals appear to display loss of concepts of territoriality following amygdalectomy, as well as changes in social status.

When the electrical activity of the amygdala is recorded, bursts of 40 per second activity are characteristically observed during states of vigilance or excited behavior (Lesse, 1960; Freeman, 1960; Adey, Dunlop and Hendrix, 1960). While such burst discharge is induced in a variety of situations, its elicitation is by no means stereotyped, but varies with the state of the animal. The presentation of food or water is evocative in deprived animals (Fig. 38), but becomes ineffective after satiety. During the establishment of a conditioned avoidance response, this burst discharge appears earlier and, in subsequent extinction, persists longer than the motor performance itself. This amygdaloid bursting is also conspicuous in approach learning but, with each attainment of the food reward, the amplitude and duration of the bursts become successively reduced (Adey, Dunlop and Hendrix, 1960). Similar patterns of high voltage, rhythmic activity have been recorded from the region of the amygdala in human sub-

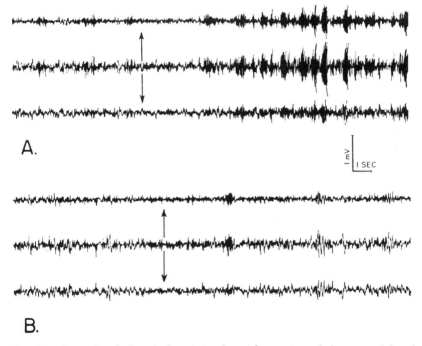

Fig. 38. Records of electrical activity from the region of the amygdala of the cat, showing the high-frequency bursts induced by fish odors in the hungry animal (A) and their virtual absence after feeding to satiety (B). From Freeman (1960).

jects during the recall of emotionally significant past experiences (Lesse, 1960).

Recent developments relating the hippocampus to memory processes involve this structure in activities beyond the visceral-regulatory and innate and emotional behavior managing capacities of the remainder of the limbic forebrain. Current views of hippocampal function may better be presented on page 135.

FOREBRAIN AND INHIBITION OF BEHAVIOR

The ready provocation of rage behavior following decortication, discussed above from the point of view of the subcortical distribution of mechanisms for its integrated performance, points as well to inhibitory influences upon such subcortical mechanisms by higher forebrain structures. Rosvold and Mishkin (1961) have recently proposed that such inhibitory deficits manifest after cerebral lesions vary with the type of activity and the neural mechanism released. An appetitive or consummatory hyperactivity occurs in the absence of inhibiting influences upon motivational systems for innate behavior. The work of Spiegel *et al.* (1940) and that of Bard and Mountcastle (1947) has indicated that injury to the limbic forebrain is the major factor leading to increased rage behavior after decortication. A similar exaggerated display of emotional behavior was observed during experimental limbic seizures (MacLean, 1958), in which mildly noxious stimuli evoked increased responsiveness leading to states of wild excitement, while enhancement of pleasure reactions might later appear.

A pronounced locomotor hyperactivity after frontal cortical lesions, referred by Ruch and Shenkin (1943) to ablation of orbito-frontal area 13, must obviously be attributed to removal of inhibition upon neural systems serving motility. In conditional reflex experiments, still another example of disinhibition following frontal lesions is provided by the repetition of trained movements hundreds of times between trials, during an experimental session (Konorski, 1961). At the same time, such frontal animals display a strong orienting reaction to the conditional signal itself, as if it were quite novel, in relation to which the performance of the trained movement is inhibited. "It is quite clear," Konorski (1961) remarks, "that what is impaired after a prefrontal lesion is only internal inhibition, while external inhibition is not affected at all or may even be increased." Rosvold and Mishkin (1961) have also noted that the frontal animal is hyperreactive and easily distracted by extraneous stimuli. Malmo (1942) has pointed out that it would be in line with the interference theory of forgetting, to suppose that the impairment of delayed response after frontal lesions should be attributed to external inhibition, associated with the orienting reflex, rather than to some more specialized deficit of recent memory itself. In keeping with this reasoning, Malmo's (1942) frontally lobectomized monkeys succeeded in delayed response performance when darkness was maintained during the period of delay but failed when the test situation was brightly lighted. Konorski (1961), on the other hand, attributes the detrimental effect of extraneous stimuli on the delayed responses of these frontal animals to their inability to "keep their bodily orientation unchanged during delay in order to perform the correct response."

Following temporal lobectomy, the repeated handling and mouthing of familiar objects, as though they were novel, as well as other symptoms described by Klüver and Bucy (1939) as visual agnosia, would also seem explicable in terms of an unchecked tendency for every signal to evoke an orienting reflex. The consequent distractibility of such animals seems most referable to ablation of the inferior temporal and entorhinal cortex, found by Adey, Segundo and Livingston (1957) to be the cortical region most potent in inhibiting ascending transmission in the brain stem reticular system. If these symptoms of heightened distractibility and perseverative exploratory behavior are attributable to a release of the orienting reflex from tempororeticular inhibition, associated external inhibition may be a factor contributing to the prevention of consolidation or recall of recent memory following temporal lobectomy, as Malmo (1942) proposed following lobectomy of the frontal cortex. Whether present after frontal or after temporal lesions, augmented external inhibition associated with the release of the orienting reflex, might prevent the consolidation or recall of recent memory at whatever focal sites in the brain this function is subserved.

There is a special relevance of the temporal lobe to memory function, however, discussion of which is deferred to page 129.

REFERENCES

Adey, W. R., Segundo, J. P. and Livingston, R. B.: Corticifugal influences on intrinsic brain stem conduction in cat and monkey. *J. Neurophysiol.*, 20:1-16, 1957.

Adey, W. R., Dunlop, C. W. and Hendrix, C. E.: Hippocampal slow waves. *AMA. Arch. Neurol.*, 3:74-90, 1960.

Andersson, B., Jewell, P. A. and Larsson, S.: An appraisal of the effects of diencephalic stimulation of conscious animals in terms of normal behavior. Pp. 76-89. In Wolstenholme, G. E. and O'Connor, V. M.: *Neurological Basis of Behavior*, Churchill, London, 1958.

Andersson, B. and McCann, S. M.: A further study of polydipsia evoked by hypothalamic stimulation in the goat. *Acta physiol. scand.*, 33: 333-346, 1955.

Anand, B. K.: Nervous regulation of food intake. *Physiol. Rev.*, 41:677-708, 1961.

Anand, B. K. and Brobeck, J. R.: Hypothalamic control of food intake in rat and cat. *Yale J. Biol. & Med.*, 24:123-140, 1951.

Bard, P. and Macht, M. B.: The behavior of chronically decerebrate cats. Pp. 55-75, In: Wolstenholme, G. E. W. and O'Connor, M. (Eds.): *The Neurological Basis of Behavior*, Churchill, London, 1958.

Bard, P. and Mountcastle, V. B.: Some forebrain mechanisms involved in expression of rage with special reference to suppression of angry behavior. *Res. Publ. Assn. Nerv. Ment. Dis.*, 27:362-404, 1947.

Bard, P. and Rioch, D. Mck.: A study of four cats deprived of neocortex and additional portions of the forebrain. *Bull. Johns Hopkins Hosp.*, 60: 73-147, 1937.

Bernard, C.: *Leçons sur les Propriétés Physiologiques et les Altérations Pathologiques des Liquides de l'Organisme.* 2 vols., Paris, 1859.

Brobeck, J. R.: Neural regulation of food intake. *Ann. New York Acad. Sc.*, 63:44-55, 1955.

Brobeck, J. R.: The internal environment and alimentary behavior. Synthesis. In: Brazier, M. A. B. (Ed.) *Brain and Behavior II*, AIBS, Washington. In press, 1962.

Broca, P.: Anatomie comparée des circonvolutions cérébrales: Le grand lobe limbique et la scissure limbique dans la série des mammiferes. *Rev. anthrop.*, 1:385-498, 1878.

Cannon, W. B.: *Wisdom of the Body*. Norton, New York, 1939.

Cross, B. A. and Green, J. D.: Activity of single neurons in the hypothalamus: effect of osmotic and other stimuli. *J. Physiol.*, 148:554-560, 1959.

Darwin, C.: *The Descent of Man and Selection in Relation to Sex.* John Murray, London, 1871.

Delgado, J. M. R., Roberts, W. W. and Miller, N. E.: Learning motivated by electrical stimulation of the brain. *Amer. J. Physiol., 179:*587-593, 1954.

Dell, P. C.: Some basic mechanisms of the translation of bodily needs into behavior. Pp. 187-203. In Wolstenholme, G. E. W. and O'Connor, C. M. (Eds.) *Neurological Basis of Behavior,* Churchill, London, 1958.

Deutsch, J. A.: *The Structural Basis of Behavior.* Univ. of Chicago Press, 1960.

Egger, M. D. and Flynn, J. P.: Amygdaloid suppression of hypothalamically elicited attack behavior. *Science, 136:*43-44, 1962.

Fernandez de Molina, A. and Hunsperger, R. W.: Central representation of affective reactions in forebrain and brain stem: electrical stimulation of amygdala, stria terminalis, and adjacent structures. *J. Physiol., 145:* 251-265, 1959.

Fernandez de Molina and Hunsperger, R. W.: Organization of subcortical system governing defense and flight reactions in the cat. *J. Physiol., 160:*200-213, 1962.

Fisher, A. E.: Maternal and sexual behavior induced by intracranial chemical stimulation. *Science, 124:*228-229, 1956.

Freeman, W. J.: Correlation of electrical activity of prepyriform cortex and behavior in cat. *J. Neurophysiol., 23:*111-131, 1960.

Fulton, J. F.: The limbic system: a study of the visceral brain in primates and man. *Yale J. Biol. Med., 26:*107-118, 1953.

Green, J. D., Clemente, C. D. and de Groot, J.: Rhinencephalic lesions and behavior in cats. *J. Comp. Neurol., 108:*505-545, 1957.

Grossman, S. P.: Eating or drinking elicited by direct adrenergic or cholinergic stimulation of hypothalamus. *Science, 132:*301-302, 1960.

Harris, G. W., Michael, R. P. and Scott, P. P.: Neurological site of action of stilbestrol in eliciting sexual behavior. Pp. 236-254. In Wolstenholme, G. E. W. and O'Connor, C. M: *Neurological Basis of Behavior.* Churchill, London, 1958.

Hervey, G. R.: The effects of lesions in the hypothalamus in parabiotic rats. *J. Physiol., 145:*336-352, 1959.

Hess, W. R.: *Diencephalon, Autonomic and Extrapyramidal Functions.* Grune and Stratton, New York, 1954.

Hetherington, A. W. and Ranson, S. W.: Hypothalamic lesions and adiposity in the rat. *Anat. Rec., 78:*149-172, 1940.

Hunsperger, R. W.: Affektreaktionen auf elektrische Reizung im Hirnstamm der Katze. *Helvet. physiol. acta, 14:*70-92, 1956.

Kaada, B. R.: Somato-motor, autonomic and electrocorticographic responses to electrical stimulation of "rhinencephalic" and other structures in primates, cat and dog. *Acta physiol. scand. (Suppl. 83),* 24:285, 1951,

Kaada, B. R., Andersen, P. and Jansen, J., Jr.: Stimulation of the amygdaloid nuclear complex in unanesthetized cats. *Neurology, 4*:48-64, 1954.

Klüver, H. and Bucy, P. C.: Preliminary analysis of functions of the temporal lobes in monkeys. *Arch. Neurol. Psychiat., 42*:979-1000, 1939.

Konorski, J.: The physiological approach to the problem of recent memory. Pp. 115-132. In Delafresnaye, J. F. (Ed.) *Brain Mechanisms and Learning,* Blackwell, Oxford, 1961.

Kubie, L. S.: Instincts and homeostasis. *Psychosom. Med., 10:*15-30, 1948.

Larsson, S.: On the hypothalamic organization of the nervous mechanism regulating food intake. Part I. *Acta physiol. scand., 32:* Suppl. 115, 1954.

Lesse, H.: Rhinencephalic electrophysiological activity during "emotional behavior" in cats. *Psychiat. Res. Rep., 12*:224-237, 1960.

Lilly, J. C.: Learning motivated by subcortical stimulation: the "start" and "stop" patterns of behavior. In Jasper, H. H. (Ed.) *Reticular Formation of the Brain.* Little, Brown, Boston, 1958.

MacLean, P. D.: Psychosomatic disease and the "visceral brain": Recent developments bearing on the Papez theory of emotion. *Psychosom. Med., 11:*338-353, 1949.

MacLean, P. D.: The limbic systems with respect to self-preservation and the preservation of the species. *J. Nerv. Ment. Dis., 127*:1-11, 1958.

MacLean, P. D.: Contrasting functions of limbic and neocortical systems of the brain and their relevance to psychophysiological aspects of medicine. *Am. J. Med., 25*:611-626, 1958.

Malmo, R. B.: Interference factors in delayed response in monkeys after removal of frontal lobes. *J. Neurophysiol., 5*:295-308, 1942.

Masserman, J. H.: *Behavior and Neurosis.* Univ. Chicago Press, 1943.

Morgane, P. J.: Medial forebrain bundle and "feeding centers" of the hypothalamus. *J. Comp. Neurol., 117*:1-25, 1961.

Olds, J.: Self-stimulation of the brain. *Science, 127*:315-324, 1958.

Olds, J. and Milner, P.: Positive reinforcement produced by electrical stimulation of septal area and other regions of rat brain. *J. Comp. Physiol. Psychol., 47*:419-427, 1954.

Papez, J. W.: A proposed mechanism of emotion. *Arch. Neurol. & Psychiat., 38*:725-745, 1937.

Pribram, K. H.: Implications for systemic studies of behavior. Chapter 39. In Sheer, D. E. (Ed.) *Electrical Stimulation of the Brain.* Univ. Texas Press, Austin, 1961.

Pribram, K. H. and Kruger, L.: Functions of the olfactory brain. *Ann. N.Y. Acad. Sci., 58*:109-138, 1954.

Richter, C. P.: Animal behavior and internal drives. *Quart. Rev. Biol., 2*:307-342, 1927.

Rosvold, H. E., Mirsky, A. F. and Pribram, K. H.: Influence of amygdalectomy on social behavior in monkeys. *J. Comp. Physiol. Psychol., 47:*173-178, 1954.

Rosvold, H. E. and Mishkin, M.: Non-sensory effects of frontal lesions on discrimination learning and performance. Pp. 555-576. In: Delafresnaye, J. F. (Ed.) *Brain Mechanisms and Learning.* Blackwell, Oxford, 1961.

Ruch, T. C. and Shenkin, H. A.: The relation of area 13 on orbital surface of frontal lobes to hyperactivity and hyperphagia in monkeys. *J. Neurophysiol., 6:*349-360, 1943.

Sawyer, C. H. and Kawakami, M.: Interactions between the central nervous system and hormones influencing ovulation. Pp. 79-97. In: Villee, C. A. (Ed.) *Control of Ovulation,* Pergamon, New York, 1961.

Schreiner, L. and Kling, A.: Behavioral changes following rhinencephalic injury in the cat. *J. Neurophysiol., 16:*643-659, 1953.

Spiegel, E. A., Miller, H. R. and Oppenheimer, M. J.: Forebrain and rage reactions. *J. Neurophysiol., 3:*538-548, 1950.

Tinbergen, N.: *The Study of Instinct.* Clarendon Press, Oxford, 1951.

Ursin, H. and Kaada, B. R.: Functional localization within the amygdaloid complex in the cat. *EEG Clin. Neurophysiol., 12:*1-20, 1960.

Wheatley, M. D.: The hypothalamus and affective behavior in cats. *Arch. Neurol. Psychiat., 52:*296-316, 1944.

Wiener, N.: *Cybernetics or Control and Communication in the Animal and Machine.* Herman & Cie, Paris, 1948.

5

RETICULO-CORTICAL INFLUENCES FOR WAKEFULNESS, ORIENTING AND ATTENTION

Having surveyed the significance of reticular influences upon spinal, brainstem and limbic activities, we may next consider the functional interrelations of the reticular system with the neocortex. It now seems clear that ascending reticular influences upon the cerebral hemispheres are importantly concerned with initiating and modifying such states as arousal and wakefulness, as well as orienting and attention. The shifting subjective aspects of these states are known to us introspectively and they can to some degree be distinguished by differences in behavior. It was not, however, until the contrasting features of sleep and wakefulness were found to be associated with differences in cortical electrical activity that progress became rapid in exploring ascending reticular influences upon higher functions of the brain.

CLASSIC CONTRIBUTIONS

Although the electroencephalogram was discovered by Caton in 1875, Beck, in 1905, was the first to observe that "its oscillations cease as soon as any one of the afferent nerves is sufficiently strongly stimulated, even though the nerve doesn't correspond at all to the cortical area examined" (Brazier, 1961). In 1913, Beck's observation was confirmed by Pravdich-Neminsky (1913) who published the first record of the EEG arousal reaction induced by peripheral stimulation (Fig. 39). In his pioneer studies, Berger (1929) noted that the EEG was composed of large slow wave-like fluctuations during sleep, while in wakefulness the record was characteristically flat. Additionally, he was the first to observe the alpha-blocking response in man.

The further contributions of Bremer (1935, 1936, 1937) and Rheinberger and Jasper (1937) laid the basis for contemporary

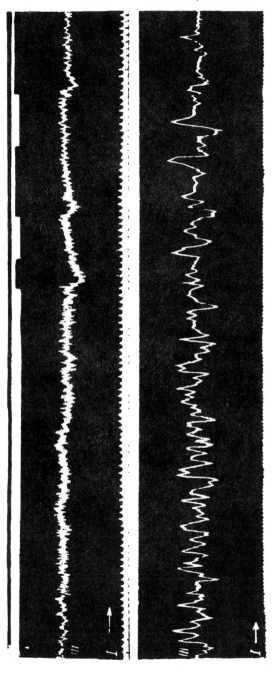

Fig. 39. The first published record of the EEG arousal reaction shows the synchronous brain potentials of a curarized dog (*above*) and the desynchronized EEG evoked by sciatic nerve stimulation (*below*). From Pravdich Neminsky (1913).

investigation. In combined EEG and behavioral study of the evocation of wakefulness by afferent stimulation in the cat, they found the low-voltage fast pattern of attentive wakefulness, termed EEG activation, to be evoked equivalently by several modalities and, however elicited, to be distributed generally over the hemisphere, without predilection for the cortical sensory area concerned. Furthermore, once initiated, this activation pattern tended to persist for long periods following the brief excitation setting it into play. Bremer (1936) pointed out: "Modification of the cortical oscillogram during passage from a state of sleep to one of wakefulness does not represent a local sensory effect of the stimulus, beginning in the cortical area corresponding to the sensory organ excited. It can be observed identically, whatever the localization of the recording electrodes, or the mode of stimulation used to awaken the animal. One is dealing here with a general modification of cortical activity."

While indicating the importance of afferent stimulation in initiating EEG and behavioral wakefulness, these observations suggested the important additional role of a central mechanism, with a more general influence and greater intrinsic capacity for maintained excitation than a specific afferent path. Bremer (1937) extended his studies to spinal and decerebrate animals and was the first to observe that the electrical activity of the cerebral hemisphere, lying *in situ* ahead of the cut, displayed a waking pattern following bulbo-spinal section while, after section through the midbrain, the record was that of sleep (Fig. 40). The behavior of portions of the head innervated from in front of the cut was in agreement and Bremer's waking *encéphale isolé* and sleeping *cerveau isolé* have since become classic preparations of neurophysiology.

ASCENDING RETICULAR SYSTEM

The program of study next to be presented has supported these basic discoveries by differentiating a corticipetal projection of the central reticular formation of the brain which subserves wakefulness and the focus of attention and through which the arousing influences of afferent stimulation are effected. In 1948, Professor G. Moruzzi, now Director of the Institute of Physiology at the University of Pisa, Italy, spent a year at Northwestern University Medical School in Chicago where, in collaborative study (1949), it was found that direct stimulation of the brain stem core reproduced all the electrocortical features observed in the EEG arousal reaction associated with natural wakefulness. In the instances illustrated in Figure 41, from subsequent experiments by Segundo, Arana-Iniguez and French (1955), reticular stimulation in monkeys with chronically implanted electrodes is seen to evoke the same pattern of low-voltage fast discharge, both in cortex and central brain stem, that is induced by peripheral afferent stimulation. These EEG alterations are further seen to coincide with behavioral awakening, depicted in frames from a motion picture. Evocation of this generalized and self-maintaining electrocortical alteration has since become commonplace, but it is still possible to recall the arousal evoked in the investigators by its initial display!

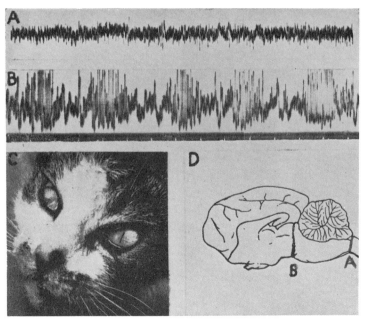

Fig. 40. Electrocorticograms of cat showing waking record (A) of *encéphale isolé* following section at bulbospinal juncture (D-A); and sleeping record (B) of *cerveau isolé* following mesencephalic section (D-B). The sleeping appearance of the latter is seen in C. From Bremer (1937).

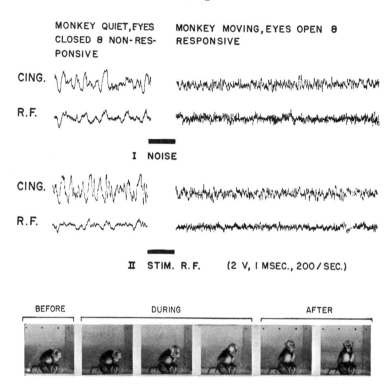

Fig. 41. Electrical activity of monkey's cingulate cortex and reticular formation, recorded with implanted electrodes (*above*), and frames from motion picture (*below*), showing EEG and behavioral arousal evoked by peripheral afferent (I) or reticular (II) stimulation. From Segundo, Arana-Iniquez and French (1955).

This electrocortical arousal could be elicited by stimulation of classical afferent paths, ascending in the periphery of the brain stem and, additionally, from its central core, comprising the reticular formation of the bulb and the tegmental portion of the pons and midbrain (Fig. 42). Within the diencephalon, the most excitable region had a paramedian distribution in the central thalamus and in the sub- and dorsal hypothalamus. Stimulating the associational thalamic nuclei was ineffective, while exciting the relay nuclei blocked slow-wave activity in the respective cortical areas to which they projected, but not generally (Starzl *et al.*, 1951). Generalized electrocortical arousal could be evoked by stimulating the non-specific thalamic nuclei, at frequencies above those yielding recruiting responses, but the lowest threshold focus lay somewhat below the intralaminar region.

It was proposed that dual routes to the cortex mediated the generalized effects: one, extra-thalamic, gaining the internal capsule directly from the subthalamic region, while the second was mediated by cortical projections of the non-specific thalamic nuclei. There now seems fair agreement that a major part of this latter projection emerges from the cephalic end of the thalamus, to reach the internal capsule through the nucleus ventralis anterior and that part of the reticular nucleus lying just in front of it (Starzl *et al.*, 1951; Hanbery *et al.*, 1953, 1954).

The significance for wakefulness of these excitable subcortical regions was next explored by observing the consequences of their experimental destruction (French and Magoun, 1952). For their two or three week periods of survival, monkeys with

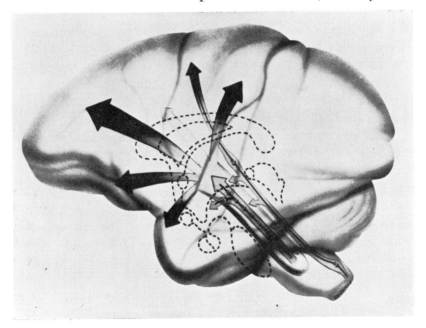

Fig. 42. Lateral view of monkey's brain, showing ascending reticular system in the core of the brain stem, receiving collaterals from an afferent pathway and projecting widely to cortical areas. From Magoun (1954).

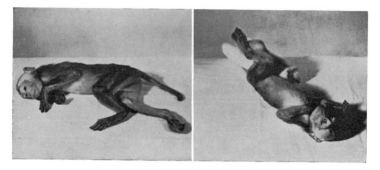

Fig. 43. Photos of a comatose monkey in the early period after lesions in the mesencephalic tegmentum and caudal diencephalon. From French and Magoun (1952).

large lesions of the central cephalic brain stem remained as though deeply asleep or anesthetized following operation (Fig. 43). Serial EEG's were composed largely of coma or stupor waves and, though the long sensory and motor paths to the cerebral cortex were spared, these animals showed no signs of awareness of their environment, nor were they capable of initiating any voluntary or purposeful movement. Neither behavioral nor EEG arousal could be evoked by the most intense afferent stimulation and, by analogy with clinical states following lesions in this same region of the brain in man (French, 1952), these animals could be described as comatose.

Conclusions from briefly surviving animals require modification, however, in the light of recent studies. Sprague, Chambers and Stellar (1961) have identified a syndrome following laterally placed midbrain lesions in the cat, in which sensory deficit, reduction of affect, hyperexploratory activity and excess oral behavior are attributed to sensory deprivation of the forebrain. Wakefulness was not impaired in these animals, however, nor was their EEG abnormal. By contrast, initial somnolence, EEG synchronization and catatonia followed more medially placed, tegmental lesions; but, after a month, these animals were easily aroused to alert wakefulness and even displayed emotional hyperexcitability to mild stimulation. Still more impressive are the preparations of Batsel (1960), who succeeded in preserving dogs for periods of months after complete mesencephalic transection.

Following the first month, the EEG of such a chronic *cerveau isolé* shifted from continuous synchronization to recurring patterns of activation, like those of wakefulness (Fig. 44). Neither the optic nor the olfactory nerves contributed essentially to this activated pattern and Batsel concluded "there is an inherent but variable tone located somewhere within the cephalic extent of the activating system, which remains connected with the cerebral cortex."

AFFERENT CONNECTIONS WITH THE RETICULAR FORMATION

The incapacity of afferent stimulation to induce EEG or be-

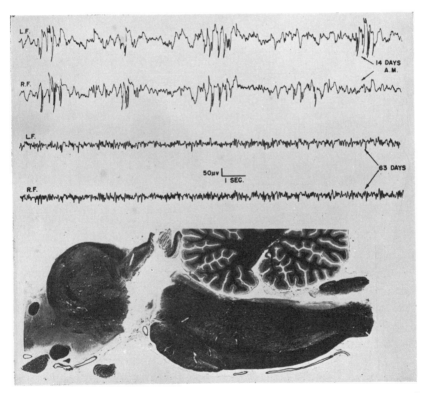

Fig. 44. Records of the frontal EEG of the dog showing a maintained synchronous pattern two weeks after (*upper*) and an asynchronous pattern two months after (*lower*), complete transection of the midbrain (*below*). From Batsel (1960).

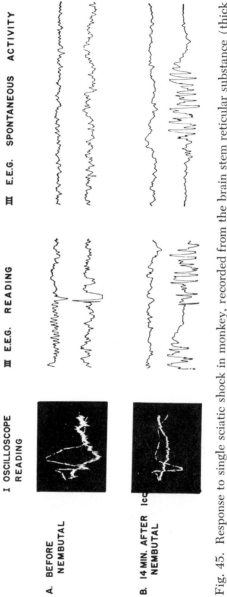

Fig. 45. Response to single sciatic shock in monkey, recorded from the brain stem reticular substance (thick beam in oscilloscope trace and upper channel of ink written record) and somatic sensory cortex (thin beam and lower channel), before and after nembutal. Note appearance of sensory afterdischarge and spindle burst in EEG after anesthesia. From French, Verzeano and Magoun (1953).

havioral arousal in the initial period after large tegmental lesions, together with its maintained effectiveness when the specific afferent paths were interrupted on each side of the midbrain (Lindsley *et al.*, 1950), suggested that peripheral arousing influences may normally be exerted through the central reticular core, rather than by impulses conveyed directly to cortical receiving areas in classical sensory paths.

The presence of such afferent connections with the reticular formation was determined by recording (Fig. 45,A) both from the core of the brain stem and from a classical afferent pathway, upon brief peripheral stimulation (Starzl *et al.*, 1951; French *et al.*, 1953). In preparations without central anesthesia, single shocks to the sciatic nerve, or clicks, evoked the customary potential changes in the classical lemniscal pathways and cortical receiving areas. Additionally, potentials with greater latency and more prolonged duration were evoked widely through the central brain stem core. It appeared that, as classical afferent paths ascended toward the cortex, collaterals passed widely from them into this central region. Responses to different modalities of stimulation could be recorded at a single reticular site and, when two stimuli of differing modality were presented in rapid succession, attenuation of the second response indicated convergence from different afferent sources upon common neural elements, with consequent lack of modality segregation.

Further evidence for afferent and other excitation of the central reticular core of the brain stem has been gained from unit studies, undertaken by the Moruzzi school at Pisa. One example, from the work of Bradley and Mollica (1958), illustrates the increased discharge of a single mesencephalic reticular unit induced by cutaneous stimulation of all four legs and face, as well as by acoustic stimuli (Fig. 46). While augmented frequency of unit firing and recruitment of quiescent elements seems most to characterize the arousal process in the brain stem, inhibition or lack of influence upon unit activity has also been observed (Machne *et al.*, 1955). Moreover, alterations in the burst-like patterns of discharge suggest the probable importance of coding in these ascending signals. In addition to afferent sources, most of the other components of the brain, including the cerebellum,

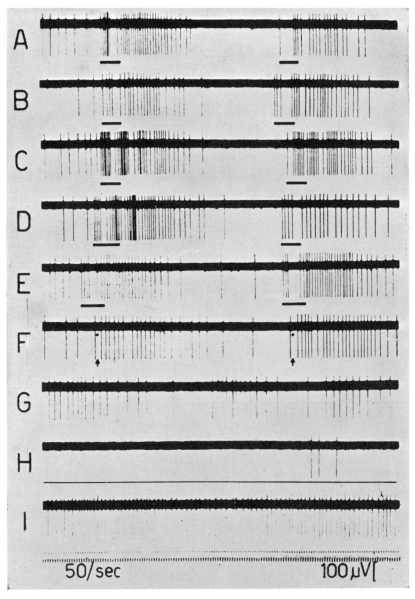

Fig. 46. Discharge of a single reticular neuron in the cat's midbrain induced by: tapping the right (A) and left (B) forelegs; the right (C) and left (D) hind legs; touching the nose (E); and click stimuli (F). Spontaneous discharge (G) is inhibited by cerebellar stimulation (H) and shows rebound excitation (I). From Bradley and Mollica (1958).

limbic system, basal ganglia and neocortex, also make functional connections with the brain stem core and are capable of influencing its performance. The manifold sources of its input, together with the multiple influences exerted by this system—cephalically upon the cortex and deep-lying mechanisms of the hemisphere, as well as caudally upon afferent relays and skeletal or visceral motor outflows from the cord—are responsible for the adjectives "non-specific" or even "indiscrete" sometimes applied to the organization and function of this portion of the brain.

RETICULAR SYSTEM AND THE ANESTHETIC STATE

While the centrally acting anesthetic agents are employed clinically to prevent pain, its loss is not a focal or differential one, as in the case of peripheral analgesia. Rather, central anesthesia is associated with loss of perception of all afferent modalities and with the disappearance of capacities for voluntary motion as well. Furthermore, in central anesthesia, afferent stimulation loses its normal capacity to evoke EEG, behavioral, and emotional arousal; and there is equivalent failure of EEG arousal upon the direct excitation of the ascending reticular system in the brain stem (Fig. 47). In the study of this phenomenon, responses evoked by afferent stimulation were recorded simultaneously from the brain stem reticular formation and from the cortical receiving area of one of the classical sensory paths. During the induction of barbiturate or ether anesthesia (French *et al.*, 1953), contrasting effects were observed, for the evoked reticular potentials were markedly reduced or abolished, while the primary, surface-positive phase of the cortical response remained unattenuated and might even be increased (Fig. 45, B). Succeeding components of this evoked response tended to be reduced or abolished, however, while sensory after-discharge appeared and spindle bursts became conspicuous. While there is no implication that the ascending reticular system is the only neural mechanism susceptible to anesthetic agents, strong evidence seems at hand that its functional and reversible block underlies the loss of consciousness in central anesthesia, as well as during such metabolic alterations as anoxia and hypoglycemia, in which unconsciousness may result (Arduini and Arduini, 1954).

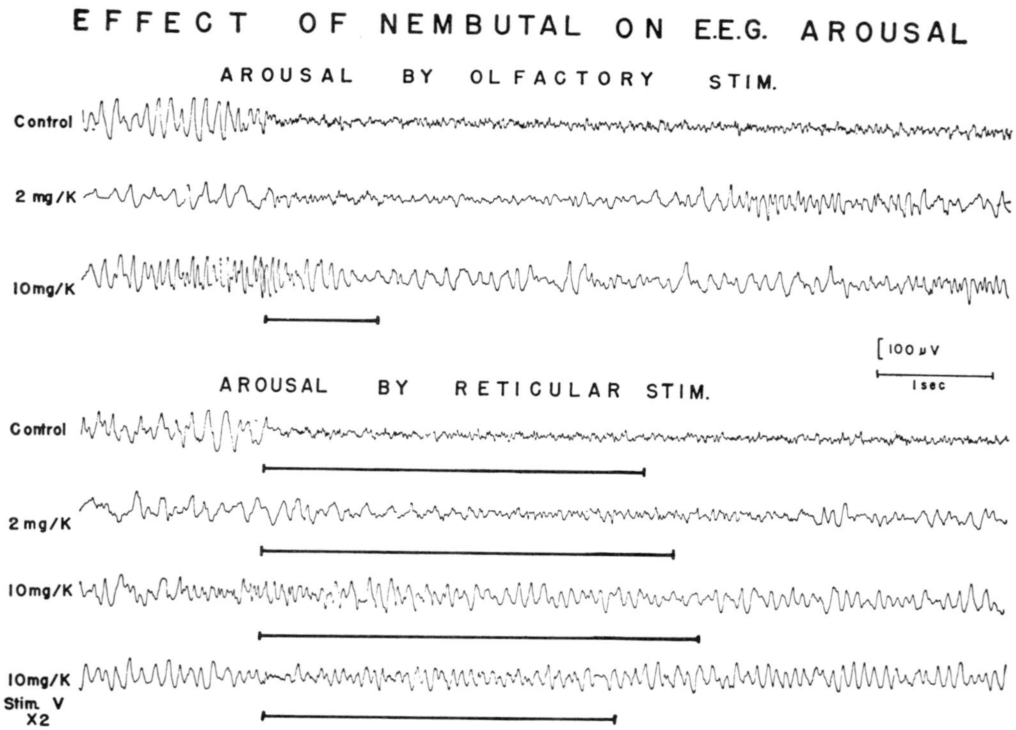

Fig. 47. Ink written records of electrocorticogram of rabbit showing effect of nembutal upon EEG arousal, induced by afferent stimulation (*above*) and direct excitation of brain stem reticular formation (*below*). From Arduini and Arduini (1954).

SPECIFICITY WITHIN THE NON-SPECIFIC SYSTEM

There is increasing indication that in spite of its ramifying interrelations, it is possible for the reticular system to subserve discriminative and differentiated, as well as generalized activities. Sharpless and Jasper (1956) have distinguished tonic and phasic levels of function in the brain stem reticular core. In the same vein, Anokhin (1961) points out that a nonspecific mechanism which invariably activated the entire hemisphere would deprive the cortex of its characteristic ability to discriminate and form selective associations. During elaboration of conditional reflexes of opposite sign, involving defensive and alimentary behavior, Anokhin has observed different types of electrical activity and, with chlorpromazin, has been able to induce differential block of responses to defensive conditional stimuli, while the animal remained awake, searched for food and ate it greedily.

RELATION TO PAIN SYSTEM

Much recent study has supported the close relationship of the pain pathway to the central reticular core. Following antero-

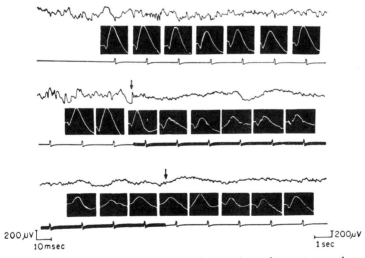

Fig. 48. Electrocorticogram of cat, with signal marking times when the dendritic (local cortical) response was evoked from the anterior suprasylvian gyrus. Note reduction of this response during EEG arousal, induced by stimulation of the brain stem between arrows. From Purpura (1956).

lateral cordotomy, both Mehler *et al.* (1960) and Bowsher (1957, 1961) have found a massive distribution of axonal degeneration within the brain stem reticular formation. Only thirty per cent of the ascending fibers continued to the diencephalon as a direct spino-thalamic tract and these appeared to be a phylogenetically recent addition, most prominent in the primates. It is proposed that this classical spino-thalamic component may contribute an immediate, sharply localized, "epicritic" quality to the appreciation of noxious stimuli; while the spino-reticular fibers and their more slowly conducting ascending relays serve the more diffusely localized, gradually developing and persistent "protopathic" features of pain sensation.

Tegmental responses evoked by peripheral nerve and tooth pulp stimulation can be readily recorded within the midbrain, where they are exceedingly sensitive to anesthetics (Collins *et al.*, 1954, 1958; Kerr, Haugen and Melzack, 1955; Haugen and Melzack, 1957; Melzack *et al.*, 1958; Spivy and Metcalf, 1959). Within the diencephalon, evidence supports the termination of the spino-thalamic tract system both in the ventrobasal and posterior complexes of the lateral thalamus (Whitlock and Perl, 1959, 1961; Perl and Whitlock, 1961; Poggio and Mountcastle, 1960; Mountcastle, 1961 a and b), as well as in the centre median, intralaminar and subthalamic regions (Albe-Fessard *et al.*, 1958, 1962; Kruger and Albe-Fessard, 1960).

It seems likely that the ascending pain pathway makes functional association in the upper brain stem with the negatively reinforcing mechanism, discussed on page 62, and it is probably in this region that the auditory masking of pain perception (Gardner *et al.*, 1960) currently applied in dental analgesia (see page 106) is to be referred. The potent arousing quality of nociceptive stimulation, related to its highly developed protective-defensive role, makes it logical that it should bear a close topographic, as well as an intimate functional relationship to the ascending reticular system.

CORTICAL CHANGES IN EEG AROUSAL

Current insight into the EEG arousal process has been gained by analysis of its modification of evoked potential or unit dis-

charges in the cortex. In a number of instances, inhibitory effects
have been observed. These include a block of chloralosane waves
and recruiting responses (Moruzzi and Magoun, 1949; Evarts
and Magoun, 1957), together with abolition of unit discharges
in the cortical motor area associated with spindle bursts or strychnine convulsive waves (Whitlock *et al.*, 1953). Similarly, the
negative component of augmenting responses is prevented (Gauthier *et al.*, 1956) and the local cortical response is reduced (Fig.
48; Purpura, 1956, 1959).

The conspicuous feature of these spindle bursts and strychnine waves, as well as recruiting, augmenting and local cortical

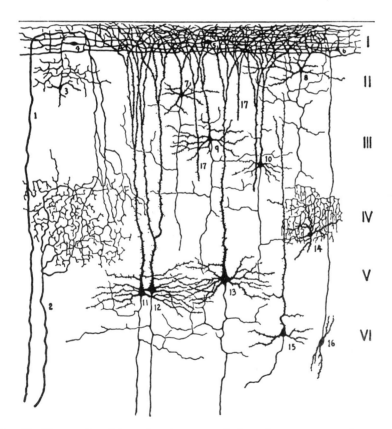

Fig. 49. Composite picture showing general plan of arrangement of neurons
in cerebral cortex, together with afferent fibers from thalamus (1 and 2,
left). From Lorente de Nó (1943).

responses, is a surface-negative deflection, with a long-time course and tendency to recruitment, now attributed to graded, non-propagating depolarization of the terminal dendritic processes of cortical pyramidal cells (Fig. 49). The generalization has recently been drawn (Bishop, 1956) of a graded response mechanism, characterizing all terminal transmitter portions of neurons, the properties of which are distinct from those of the intervening conducting axone, where depolarization is brief, all-or-none, and followed by refractoriness. Purpura (1956, 1959) has concluded that EEG arousal is primarily associated with an inhibition of such graded dendritic activity.

Since practically all higher neural activity occurs during wakefulness, rather than in sleep, it might be presumed that EEG arousal should favor rather than reduce some features of cortical excitability and performance. During experimental reticular stimulation, visual discrimination is improved (Fuster, 1958) and the recovery cycle of the optic cortex has been found to be reduced (Lindsley, 1958, 1961). Moreover, the motor cortex is more excitable during wakefulness, as compared with drowsiness or sleep (Lilly, 1958). A focal flattening of the EEG, recorded from the motor cortex, is associated with initiation of voluntary type movements in both the monkey (Kruger and Henry, 1957) and man (Penfield and Jasper, 1954). These observations suggest that cortical excitability may be improved, rather than reduced, during EEG arousal.

In agreement, Bremer and Stoupel (1959) and Dumont and Dell (1960) have recently demonstrated dramatic reticular facilitation of responses induced in the visual, auditory or somatic cortical areas by appropriate thalamic stimulation (Figs. 50, 60). Both the initial positive and succeeding negative phases of these evoked responses were augmented. Increase of the positive phase was preserved after focal pentobarbital block of the negative component, suggesting that facilitation is operative both at somal and dendritic sites. From these findings, both facilitatory and inactivating influences from the central brain stem contribute importantly to the cortical state upon which most higher nervous activity depends.

Steady potential changes, in which the surface of the cortex shifts negative to a reference electrode (Fig. 51), are regularly induced by reticular and thalamic stimulation (Arduini *et al.,* 1957; Brookhart *et al.,* 1958; Vanasupa *et al.,* 1959). Their distribution is focal or generalized, depending upon the input involved. They have been attributed to sustained post-synaptic depolarization of the same neuronal elements responsible for the surface-negative components of recruiting or augmenting responses. In the behaving animal, Caspers (1961) has observed that evocation of such cortical negativity "corresponds to the general attention reaction and gradually decreases in amplitude and duration as the animal becomes habituated to the laboratory milieu." Provoked arousal and orientation are accompanied by steeper negative shifts, the maximal deflection corresponding to the peak of EEG arousal, with gradual return to a mean level of wakefulness. During sleep, contrastingly, the cortical steady potential shifts toward the positive side. These alterations during the sleep-wakefulness cycle suggest the relation of steady potentials to changes in cortical excitability (Brazier, 1962).

Recent studies of single neuron activity have identified an alteration in pattern, rather than a change in rate of unit firing,

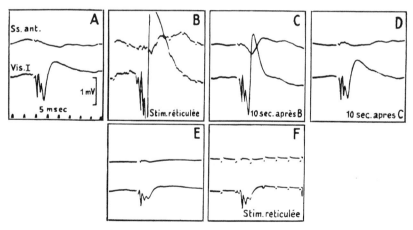

Fig. 50. Records showing the pronounced facilitation of all phases of the visual cortical response to optic nerve shocks (A), induced by reticular stimulation (B). Facilitation is declining at ten seconds (C) and absent after twenty seconds (D). The effect is abolished by barbiturate anesthesia (E, F). From Bremer and Stoupel (1959).

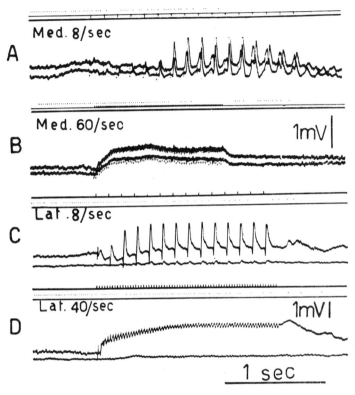

Fig. 51. Records showing steady potential changes (cortical negativity), accompanying recruiting responses (A), augmenting responses (C), and EEG arousal reactions (B and D), evoked by thalamic stimulation in the cat. From Brookhart, Arduini, Mancia and Moruzzi (1958).

as a characteristic difference between sleep and wakefulness (Creutzfeldt and Jung, 1961). During sleep, grouped discharges of adjacent neurons recurred in rhythmic bursts while, with arousal, this intermittent pattern of firing changed to more or less continuous discharge. Hubel (1959) also noted that bursts were smoothed out during arousal, giving a marked increase in firing regularity. These changes in cortical neuronal activity are seen to advantage in contrasting firing patterns of pyramidal tract units during synchronization and desynchronization of the motor cortical EEG (Calma and Arduini, 1954). In addition, Evarts (1960, 1961) has pointed out that waking is associated with a reduction of spontaneous discharge in the majority of cortical units, with a corresponding increase in the ratio of evoked activity. This greater degree of differentiation within cellular populations, he suggests, may serve to heighten sensitivity during wakefulness.

REFERENCES

Albe-Fessard, D. and Kruger, L.: Duality of unit discharge from cat centrum medianum in response to natural and electrical stimulation. *J. Neurophysiol.*, 25:3-20, 1962.

Albe-Fessard, D. and Rougeul, A.: Activités d'origine somesthétique évoquées sur le cortex non-spécifique du chat anesthésié au chloralose: Rôle du centre médian du thalamus. *EEG Clin. Neurophysiol.*, 10: 131-152, 1958.

Anokhin, P. K.: The multiple ascending influences of the subcortical centers on the cerebral cortex, pp. 139-170. In Brazier, M. A. B. (Ed.)*Brain and Behavior I*, AIBS, Washington, 1961.

Arduini, A. and Arduini, M. G.: Effect of drugs and metabolic alterations on brain stem arousal mechanism. *J. Pharmacol. & Exper. Therap.*, 110: 76-85, 1954.

Arduini, A., Mancia, M. and Mechelse, K.: Slow potential changes in the cerebral cortex by sensory and reticular stimulation. *Arch. ital. Biol.*, 95: 127-138, 1957.

Batsel, H. L.: Electroencephalographic synchronization and desynchronization in the chronic "cerveau isolé" in the dog. *EEG clin. Neurophysiol.*, 12:421-430, 1960.

Berger, H.: Uber das Elektrenkephalogramm des Menschen. *Arch. f. Psychiat.*, 87:527-570, 1929.

Bishop, G. H.: Natural history of the nerve impulse. *Physiol. Rev., 36*: 376-399, 1956.

Bowsher, D.: Termination of the central pain pathway in man; the conscious appreciation of pain. *Brain, 80*:606-622, 1957.

Bowsher, D.: The termination of secondary somatosensory neurones within the thalamus of Macaca Mulatta: An experimental degeneration study. *J. comp. Neurol.*, 117:213-227, 1961.

Bowsher, D.: The reticular formation and ascending reticular system: anatomical considerations. *Brit. J. Anaesth, 33*:174-182, 1961.

Bradley, P. B. and Mollica, A.: The effect of adrenaline and acetylcholine on single unit activity in the reticular formation of the decerebrate cat. *Arch. ital. Biol.*, 96:168-186, 1958.

Brazier, M. A. B.: *A History of the Electrical Activity of the Brain*, Pitman, London, 1961.

Brazier, M. A. B. (Ed.) *Brain Function and Space Science I. Steady Potentials and Cortical Excitability.* AIBS, Washington, In press, 1962.

Bremer, F.: Cerveau isolé et physiologie du sommeil. *C. R. Soc. Biol.* (Paris), *118*:1235-1242, 1935.

Bremer, F.: Nouvelles recherches sur le mécanisme du sommeil. *C. R. Soc. Biol.* (Paris), *122*:460-464, 1936.

Bremer, F.: Activité électrique du cortex cérébral dans les états de sommeil et de veille chez le chat. *L. R. Soc. Biol.* (Paris), *122*:464-467, 1936.

Bremer, F.: L'activité cérébrale au cours du sommeil et de la narcose. Contribution à l'étude du mécanisme du sommeil. *Bull. Acad. Roy. Med., Belgique, 2*:68-86, 1937.

Bremer, F. and Terzuolo, C.: Contribution à l'étude des mécanismes physiologiques du maintien de l'activité vigile du cerveau. Interaction de la formation réticulée et de l'écorce cérébrale dans le processus du réveil. *Arch. internat. physiol., 62*:157-178, 1954.

Bremer, F. and Stoupel, N.: Facilitation et inhibition des potentials évoqués corticaux dans l'éveil cérébral. *Arch. internat. Physiol., 67*:240-275, 1959.

Brookhart, J. M., Arduini, A., Mancia, M. and Moruzzi, G.: Thalamocortical relations as revealed by induced slow potential changes. *J. Neurophysiol., 21*:499-525, 1958.

Calma, I. and Arduini, A.: Spontaneous and induced activity in pyramidal units. *J. Neurophysiol., 17*:321-335, 1954.

Casper, H.: Changes of cortical D.C. potentials in the sleep-wakefulness cycle, pp. 237-259. In Wolstenholme, G. E. W. and O'Connor, M. (Eds.) *The Nature of Sleep,* Churchill, London, 1961.

Collins, W. F. and O'Leary, J. L.: Study of a somatic evoked response of midbrain reticular substance. *EEG clin. Neurophysiol., 6*:619-628, 1954.

Collins, W. F. and Randt, C. T.: Evoked central nervous system activity relating to peripheral unmyelinated or "C" fibers in cat. *J. Neurophysiol., 21*:345-352, 1958.

Creutzfeldt, O. and Jung, R.: Neuronal discharge in the cat's motor cortex during sleep and arousal, pp. 131-170, in Wolstenholme, G. E. W. and O'Connor, M. (Eds.) *The Nature of Sleep,* Churchill, London, 1961.

Dumont, S. and Dell, P.: Facilitation réticulaire des mécanismes visuels corticaux. *EEG Clin. Neurophysiol., 12*:769-796, 1960.

Evarts, E. V.: Effects of sleep and waking on spontaneous and evoked discharge of single units in visual cortex. *Fed. Proc., 19*:828-837, 1960.

Evarts, E. V.: Effects of sleep and waking on activity of single units in the unrestrained cat, pp. 171-182. In Wolstenholme, G. E. W. and O'Connor, M. (Eds.) *The Nature of Sleep,* Churchill, London, 1961.

Evarts, E. V. and Magoun, H. W.: Some characteristics of cortical recruiting responses in unanesthetized cats. *Science, 125*:1147-1148, 1957.

French, J. D.: Brain lesions associated with prolonged unconsciousness. *Arch. Neurol. & Psychiat., 68*:727-740, 1952.

French, J. D. and Magoun, H. W.: Effects of chronic lesions in central cephalic brain stem of monkeys. *Arch. Neurol. & Psychiat., 68*:591-604, 1952.

French, J. D., Verzeano, M. and Magoun, H. W.: An extralemniscal sensory system in the brain. *Arch. Neurol. & Psychiat., 69*:505-518, 1953.

French, J. D., Verzeano, M. and Magoun, H. W.: A neural basis for the anesthetic state. *Arch. Neurol. & Psychiat., 69*:519-529, 1953.

Fuster, J. M.: Effects of stimulation of brain stem on tachistoscopic perception. *Science, 127*:150, 1958.

Gardner, W. J., Licklider, J. C. R. and Weisz, A. Z.: Suppression of pain by sound. *Science, 132*:32-33, 1960.

Gauthier, C., Parma, M. and Zanchetti, A.: Effect of electrocortical arousal upon development and configuration of specific evoked potentials. *EEG Clin. Neurophysiol., 8*:237-243, 1956.

Hanberry, J., Ajmone-Marsan, C. and Dilworth, M.: Pathways of non-specific thalamo-cortical projection system. *EEG Clin. Neurophysiol., 6*:103-118, 1954.

Hanberry, J. and Jasper, H. H.: Independence of diffuse thalamocortical projection system shown by specific nuclear destruction. *J. Neurophysiol., 16*:252-271, 1953.

Haugen, F. P. and Melzack, R.: The effects of nitrous oxide on responses evoked in the brain stem by tooth stimulation. *Anesthesiology, 18*: 183-195, 1957.

Hubel, D. W.: Single unit activity in striate cortex of unrestrained cats. *J. Physiol., 147*:226-238, 1959.

Kerr, D. B., Haugen, F. and Melzack, R.: Responses evoked in brain stem by tooth stimulation. *Am. J. Physiol., 183*:253-258, 1955.

Kruger, L. and Henry, C. E.: The electrical activity of the Rolandic region in the unanesthetized monkey. *Neurology, 7*:490-495, 1957.

Kruger, L. and Albe-Fessard, D.: Distribution of responses to somatic afferent stimuli in the diencephalon of the cat under chloralose anesthesia. *Exp. Neurol., 2*:442-467, 1960.

Lilly, J.: Correlations between neurophysiological activity in the cortex and short-term behavior in the monkey. *Interdisciplinary Research Symposium,* Univ. Wisconsin Press, Madison, 1958.

Lindsley, D. B., Schreiner, L. H., Knowles, W. B. and Magoun, H. W.: Behavioral and EEG changes following chronic brain stem lesions in the cat. *EEG Clin. Neurophysiol., 2*:483-498, 1950.

Lindsley, D. B.: The reticular system and perceptual discrimination, pp. 513-534. In Jasper, H. H. (Ed.) *Reticular Formation of the Brain.* Little Brown, Boston, 1958.

Lindsley, D. B.: Electrophysiology of the visual system and its relation to perceptual phenomena, pp. 359-392. In Brazier, M. A. B. (Ed.) *Brain and Behavior I,* AIBS, Washington, 1961.

Lorente de Nó, R.: Cerebral cortex: architecture, intracortical connections, motor projections. In: Fulton, J. F., *Physiology of the Nervous System,* Oxford University Press, 1943.

Machne, X., Calma, I. and Magoun, H. W.: Unit activity of central cephalic brain stem in EEG arousal. *J. Neurophysiol., 18*:547-558, 1955.

Magoun, H. W.: The ascending reticular system and wakefulness, pp. 1-20. In Delafresnaye, J. F. (Ed.) *Brain Mechanisms and Consciousness,* Blackwell, Oxford, 1954.

Mehler, W. H., Feferman, M. E. and Nauta, W. J. H.: Ascending axon degeneration following anterolateral cordotomy. An experimental study in the monkey. *Brain, 83*:718-750, 1960.

Melzack, R., Stotler, W. A. and Livingston, W. K.: Effects of discrete brain-stem lesions in cats on perception of noxious stimulation. *J. Neurophysiol., 21*:353-367, 1958.

Moruzzi, G. and Magoun, H. W.: Brain stem reticular formation and activation of the EEG. *EEG Clin. Neurophysiol., 1*:455-473, 1949.

Mountcastle, V. B.: Some functional properties of the somatic afferent system, pp. 403-436. In Rosenblith, W. (Ed.) *Sensory Communication.* M.I.T., Wiley, New York, 1961.

Mountcastle, V. B.: Duality of function in the somatic afferent system, pp. 67-93. In Brazier, M. A. B. (Ed.) *Brain and Behavior I,* AIBS, Washington, 1961.

Penfield, W. and Jasper, H. H.: *Epilepsy and the Functional Anatomy of the Human Brain,* Little Brown, Boston, 1954.

Perl, E. R. and Whitlock, D. G.: Somatic stimuli exciting spinothalamic projections to thalamic neurons in cat and monkey. *Exper. Neurol., 3*: 256-296, 1961.

Poggio, G. F. and Mountcastle, V. B.: A study of the functional contributions of the lemniscal and spinothalamic systems to somatic sensibility, central nervous mechanism in pain. *Bull. Johns Hopk. Hosp., 106*:266-316, 1960.

Pravdich-Neminsky, V. V.: Ein Versuch der Registrierung der elektrischen Gehirnerscheinungen. *Zbl. Physiol., 27*:951-960, 1913.

Purpura, D. P.: Observations on the cortical mechanisms of EEG activation accompanying behavioral arousal. *Science, 123*:804, 1956.

Purpura, D. P.: Nature of electrocortical potentials and synaptic organizations in cerebral and cerebellar cortex. *Internat. Rev. Neurobiol., 1*: 47-163, Academic Press, New York, 1959.

Segundo, J. P., Arana-Iniquez, R. and French, J. D.: Behavioral arousal by stimulation of the brain in the monkey. *J. Neurosurg., 12*:601-613, 1955.

Sharpless, S. and Jasper, H. H.: Habituation of the arousal reaction. *Brain, 79*:655-680, 1956.

Spivy, D. F. and Metcalf, J. S.: Differential effects of medial and lateral dorsal root sections upon subcortical evoked potentials. *J. Neurophysiol., 22*:367-373, 1959.

Sprague, J. M., Chambers, W. W. and Stellar, E.: Attentive, affective and adaptive behavior in the cat. *Science, 133:*165-173, 1961.

Starzl, T. E. and Magoun, H. W.: Organization of the diffuse thalamic projection system. *J. Neurophysiol., 14:*133-146, 1951.

Starzl, T. E., Taylor, C. W. and Magoun, H. W.: Ascending conduction in the reticular activating system with special reference to the diencephalon. *J. Neurophysiol., 14:*461-477, 1951.

Starzl, T. E., Taylor, C. W. and Magoun, H. W.: Collateral afferent excitation of reticular formation of brain stem. *J. Neurophysiol., 14:*479-496, 1951.

Vanasupa, P., Goldring, S., O'Leary, J. L. and Winter, D.: Steady potential changes during cortical activation. *J. Neurophysiol., 22:*273-284, 1959.

Whitlock, D. G., Arduini, A. and Moruzzi, G.: Microelectrode analysis of pyramidal system during transition from sleep to wakefulness. *J. Neurophysiol., 16:*414-429, 1953.

Whitlock, D. G. and Perl, E. R.: Afferent projections through ventrolateral funiculi to thalamus of cat. *J. Neurophysiol., 22:*133-148, 1959.

Whitlock, D. G. and Perl, E. R.: Thalamic projections of spinothalamic pathways in monkey. *Exper. Neurol., 3:*240-255, 1961.

6

CORTICO-RETICULAR RELATIONS

WHILE INITIAL STUDY of the reticular system and wakefulness dealt chiefly with ascending influence upon the cortex, much recent attention has been directed to reciprocal influences exerted by the cortex upon the central brain stem core. A number of cortical regions have been found to project to the reticular system (Jasper *et al.*, 1952; French *et al.*, 1955) and their collective magnitude is second only to that from peripheral receptors. Generalized EEG arousal and behavioral wakefulness can be induced by exciting these cortico-reticular projections (Fig. 52; Bremer and Terzuolo, 1953), more especially those arising from

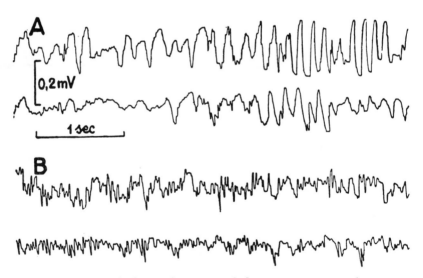

Fig. 52. Records of electrical activity of the posterior suprasylvian gyrus and auditory area of the left hemisphere of an *encéphale isolé*, with section of the corpus callosum: (A), during sleep and (B), during EEG arousal provoked by brief stimulation of the right paravisual cortex. From Bremer and Terzuolo (1953).

the cingulate, orbital and lateral frontal regions, central and para-occipital areas, and the superior gyrus and tip of the temporal lobe (Fig. 53; French, Hernandez-Péon, and Livingston, 1955; Kaada and Johannessen, 1960; Fengel and Kaada, 1960). Their facilitatory and other interactions with activity in the reticular system have been shown by Adey, Segundo and Livingston (1957). EEG patterns of wakefulness observed in the chronic *cerveau isolé* (Fig. 44) may depend upon recovery in these functional circuits between cortical regions and the diencephalic reticular system (Batsel, 1960).

Such cortico-reticular influences are capable of reducing, as well as augmenting the excitability of the central brain stem core. In ingenious experiments, Hugelin and Bonvallet (1957) have observed midbrain reticular facilitation of serially repeated spinal reflexes in preparations with intact cortex and following decortication (Fig. 54). With cortical function eliminated, reticular facilitation of reflex responses persisted throughout the period of midbrain stimulation. In the intact brain, by contrast, when the cortical EEG arousal reaction was evoked by midbrain stimulation, initial facilitation of the spinal reflex gave way to its succeeding inhibition. Hugelin and Bonvallet propose that, as reticular stimulation begins to facilitate performance, both at cortical and lower reflex levels, it sets into play an inverse, inhibitory, cortico-reticular feedback, which checks excitation and so turns down the gain of the reticulo-cortical influences

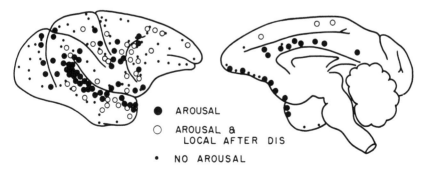

● AROUSAL

○ AROUSAL & LOCAL AFTER DIS

∙ NO AROUSAL

Fig. 53. Lateral and medial aspects of monkey's cortex, with circles marking sites whose stimulation evoked generalized EEG arousal. From Segundo, Naquet and Buser (1955).

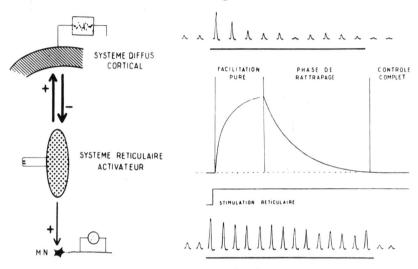

Fig. 54. Records and graph at *upper right* show facilitation of successive spinal reflex discharge by midbrain reticular stimulation. As cortical excitability is concomitantly elevated, a negative cortico-reticular feedback reduces reticular excitability, marked by decline or loss of reflex facilitation (*see schema at left*). After decortication (*lower record at right*), reticulospinal facilitation is no longer reduced. From Hugelin and Bonvallet (1957).

setting it into play. These findings indicate that the reticular system does not normally facilitate activity without provision for self-regulatory control. They advance an homeostatic role served by inverse feedbacks promoting stability and preventing over-activity and over-responsiveness of the brain.

CENTRIFUGAL CONTROL OF AFFERENT FUNCTION

One of the most significant examples of this principle of homeostasis in reticular function has come from the demonstration of its feedback control of inputs to the CNS. The model of central management of proprioceptive input from the muscle spindle, through its gamma motor regulation, developed by Granit (1955) and discussed above (page 33), led Hagbarth and Kerr (1954) to explore the possibility that the reticular system might more generally influence the excitability of somatic afferent relays within the spinal cord.

When the effects of reticular stimulation were tested upon ascending dorsal column volleys, evoked by single shock stimuli to a lumbar dorsal root (Fig. 55), the direct fiber response was found to be unaffected, while all post-synaptic activities—including the relayed posterior column response, the dorsal root reflex and all but the initial phase of the intermediary cord potential—were greatly attenuated or abolished. Relayed activity ascending in the ventral column of the cord was similarly reduced or prevented by reticular stimulation, whether by direct excitation of the central brain stem core or inputs to it from the cerebral cortex or cerebellum. This inhibitory influence appears to be a tonic one (Fig. 56), for a minimal ventral column response to dorsal root shocks is markedly increased in amplitude after eliminating influences from the brain by high spinal transection (Lindbloom and Ottosson, 1953; Hagbarth and Kerr, 1954). Unlike the bivalency of reticular influences on lower motor mechanisms, only inhibitory reticulo-spinal control appears to be exerted at lower afferent relays although, as discussed on page 90, facilitation of afferent responses in the cortex has recently been observed.

Succeeding study by Hernandez-Péon (1955, 1960, 1961) has demonstrated comparable reticular influences upon afferent transmission in the posterior column nuclei, as well as in trigeminal and cochlear nuclei of the bulb. Similar centrifugal effects have been observed upon cochlear nuclear and retinal activity, and analogous influences are exerted at the olfactory bulb by centrifugal fibers of the anterior commissure. Modulating influences have thus been identified in each of the major sensory systems. Hernandez-Péon (1961) has drawn the generalization that "the reticular mechanisms of sensory filtering are formed by feedback loops, with an ascending segment from second-order sensory neurons to the reticular formation and a descending limb in the opposite direction (Fig. 57). Such an arrangement prevents overactivation of sensory neurons and, therefore, an excessive bombardment of the brain by afferent impulses. Their exclusion takes place at the entrance gates of the central nervous system. The first sensory synapse functions as a valve where sensory filtering occurs."

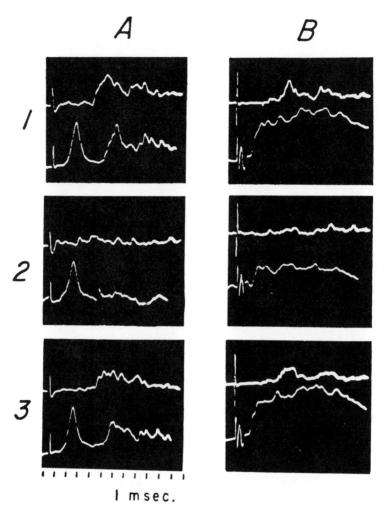

A

B

1

2

3

I msec.

Fig. 55. Effect of bulbo-reticular stimulation upon cord responses to single shock stimulus of L7 dorsal root of cat. A. Dorsal root reflex (*upper beam*) and dorsal column response (*lower beam*), before (1), during (2), and after (3) reticular stimulation. B. Dorsal root reflex (*upper*) and negative intermediary potential (*lower beam*) recorded from the dorsal root entry zone, before (1), during (2), and after (3) reticular stimulation. From Hagbarth and Kerr (1954).

A number of studies have stressed an additional feedback control of input exerted at peripheral receptors themselves. Central regulation of cochlear excitability through changing tension of the middle-ear muscles has been demonstrated by Hugelin *et al.* (1960). Analogous central control of retinal discharge, by modification of the pupillary aperture, has been shown by Naquet *et al.* (1960) and by Fernandez-Guardiola *et al* (1961). It is now additionally clear that corticifugal control of sensory input can be effected by the pyramidal tract, as well as by reticular mechanisms. In degeneration studies, Kuypers (1960) has found pyramidal tract terminals in the spinal trigeminal complex, the posterior column nuclei and the posterior horn of the spinal cord. Striking modification of afferent transmission through the posterior column nuclei, by pyramidal tract excitation, has recently been demonstrated by Towe and Jabbur (1960) and Guzman Flores *et al.* (1962).

AFFERENT CONDUCTION DURING FOCUS OF ATTENTION

The feedback control of input by the reticular system may serve to prevent the intrusion into consciousness of information

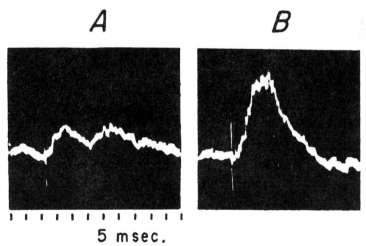

Fig. 56. Oscilloscope records of ventral column response to stimulation of lumbar dorsal root in cat, before (A) and one hour after (B) high spinal transection. From Hagbarth and Kerr (1954).

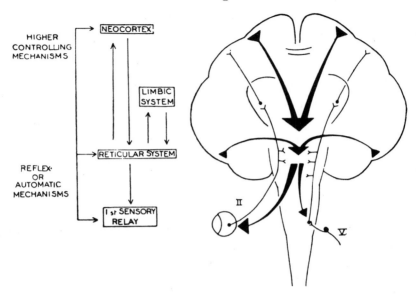

Fig. 57. Diagrammatic representation of mechanisms regulating sensory inflow to the brain. For simplicity, only the afferent visual and trigeminal pathways are shown. Corticifugal feedbacks to sensory relays and reticular formation are seen in heavy black. From Hernandez-Péon (1961).

irrelevant to the task at hand, and so contribute to the focus of attention. Hernandez-Péon, Scherrer and Jouvet (1956) have recorded the response of the cat's cochlear nucleus to click stimuli presented repetitively. They found prominent potentials, evoked in the relaxed or drowsing state, to be attenuated markedly when the animal's behavior was attracted visually by mice presented in a beaker (Fig. 58). When the mice were removed, and the cat drowsed again, the click-evoked cochlear nuclear responses resumed initial amplitude. Similar attenuation of repetitively evoked auditory or tactile responses occurred when the cat's attention was attracted by olfactory stimulation from fish odors, blown into its cage through a tube.

The circumscription of the field of awareness, which is so important in the focus of attention, would appear from these observations to depend, at least in part, upon the active exclusion of irrelevant information, so as to prevent its passage farther into the central nervous system than the first synapse in the afferent path. To a degree, these events resemble the still more focal changes during excitation in classical sensory systems. During illumination of the retina (Kuffler, 1952), central excitation is accompanied by an active reduction of discharge in the surrounding peripheral field. A similar principle appears operative in the somatic receiving cortex, and "this pattern of central excitation and surround inhibition of the receptive fields, appears to be a basic one for many afferent systems" (Mountcastle, 1961).

CLICK RESPONSES
IN COCHLEAR NUCLEUS

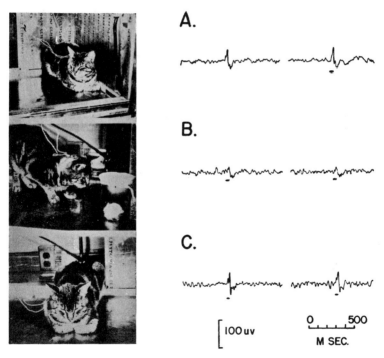

Fig. 58. Ink written records of response of cochlear nucleus to serially repeated clicks, when cat is inattentive (A), when its attention is attracted by mice in a beaker (B), and when it is inattentive again (C). From Hernandez-Péon, Scherrer and Jouvet (1956).

The more general features of such sensory interaction and control are now gaining practical application in the masking of pain by sound in clinical dentistry. The patient wears headphones and himself regulates the intensity both of stereophonic music and of white noise. The main function of the music is to relax the patient before the painful stage. When pain is anticipated or begins, the patient turns up the intensity of noise stimulation and so drowns out the pain. Several factors operate simultaneously in producing this audioanalgesia. According to Gardner *et al.* (1960), "the noise appears in introspection directly to suppress the pain. It also masks the sound of the dental drill, thereby removing a source of conditioned anxiety. The music promotes relaxation and the noise, which sounds like a waterfall, also has a relaxing effect. When both are presented, the music can be followed only through concentration, which diverts attention from the dental operation. Suggestion also plays a role, the significance of which has been difficult to estimate."

HABITUATION

In another category of feedback control of input, cortico-reticular systems reduce or prevent central neural involvement by inconsequential, stereotyped, monotonously-repeated stimulation. A classic paper on such habituation by Sharpless and Jasper (1956) opens with the lines, "If a drop of water falls on the surface of the sea, just over the flower-like disc of a sea-anemone, the whole animal contracts vigorously. If then, a second drop falls within a few minutes of the first, there is less contraction, and finally, on the third or fourth drop, the response disappears altogether. Here, in this marine polyp, is clearly exhibited one of the most pervasive phenomena of the animal kingdom—decrement of response with repeated stimulation."

A typical pattern of habituation of the arousal reaction in the cat (Fig. 59) starts with the prolonged evocation of EEG arousal upon the initial presentation of a brief 500 cycle tone (Sharpless and Jasper, 1956). With its recurring presentation, the duration of the evoked activation becomes progressively reduced until, on the thirty-sixth trial, it is limited to the period of the stimulus. On the thirty-seventh trial, the arousal reaction no longer occurs at all and is said to be habituated. This habituation is not the result of fatigue or other generalized impairment of the arousal mechanism for, in succeeding trials, tones of different pitch again evoke a full-blown response. Although the process obviously displays specificity, in the sense that it must involve neural mechanisms capable of pitch discrimination, such habituation can still be established after bilateral ablation of auditory areas I and II. Additionally, the feedback mechanism involved differs from that in the focus of attention, in which factors relating to EEG arousal exclude irrelevant information. In habituation, conversely, the monotonous presentation of irrelevant information excludes the EEG arousal reaction. This consequence cannot be attributed to block of input at lower sensory relays for, during habituation, auditory responses continue to be evoked in the cortex without reduction of amplitude (Sharpless and Jasper, 1956).

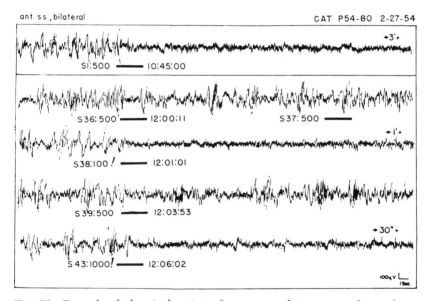

Fig. 59. Records of electrical activity from suprasylvian gyrus of cat, showing habituation of arousal reaction to 500 cycle tone (heavy bar below record), the number of presentations of which are designated by S 1, S 36, etc. (at the times indicated). Note habituation to 500 cycle tone on 37th and 39th trials, with marked arousal to novel, 100 and 1000 cycle tones in same period. From Sharpless and Jasper (1956).

SENSORY DEPRIVATION

Current interest in sensory deprivation (Solomon, 1961), stems from the manifold instances in industry, defense and other preoccupations of contemporary civilization in which individuals, subjected to monotonous situations for long periods, display reduction of attention leading to impaired performance. Additionally, sensory deprivation provides an experimental means of induction and study of some of the symptoms which characterize types of mental illness. Among the procedures employed, the provision of exteroceptive contacts of a neutral, unvaried type; the supply of a stable masking sound to the ear; and the presentation of a steady, unpatterned, translucent light to the eye; all suggest that afferent stimulation is not eliminated, as the term deprivation implies, but rather is maintained in a monotonous fashion promoting habituation. When prolonged, such monotonous input to the CNS leads to anxiety, motor restlessness, distortions of perception and, sometimes, hallucinations.

The field of study of the role of sensory and more general experiential, social, and cultural deprivation during the early years of life, upon subsequent development and capability, is now coming widely to attention for its relevance to education and the etiology of mental retardation. The situation today is not unlike that in philosophy in the seventeenth and eighteenth centuries, when the importance of sensation in producing ideas in the mind first began to receive modern formulation. John Locke inaugurated "sensationalism" in his *Essay Concerning Human Understanding* (1690), when he wrote "If we suppose the mind to be white paper void of all characters, without any ideas, whence comes it by that vast store which the busy and boundless fancy of man has painted on it with an almost endless variety? To this I answer, in two words, 'from experience.' In that, all our knowledge is founded. If a child were kept in a place where he never saw any other colors but black or white till he was man, he would have no more idea of scarlet or green than he that from his childhood never tasted an oyster or a pineapple, has of these particular relishes."

ORIENTING REFLEX

With the growing exchange of scientific information between Soviet and Western physiology, it has become clear that the arousal reaction of recent Western study is identical with, or forms a part of the Pavlovian orienting or investigatory reflex (Voronin and Sokolov, 1960; Sokolov, 1960; Razran, 1961; John, 1961). In Pavlov's (1927) original description, "the appearance of any new stimulus immediately evokes the investigatory reflex and the animal fixes all its appropriate receptor organs upon the source of disturbance, pricking up its ears, fastening its gaze upon the disturbing agency and sniffing the air." In more recent elaboration, in addition to the generalized EEG arousal reaction, the orienting reflex includes somatic, visceral and other central neural alterations, all of which tend to enhance the discriminatory power of the analyzers, enabling them to gain more information about the evocative stimulus, toward which the eyes, head and body are oriented (Fig. 60; Dumont and Dell, 1960). There are usually also changes in respiration and heartbeat, along with vasodilation of the head vessels, vasoconstriction of the finger vessels and a galvanic skin response.

The orienting reflex differs from adaptive reflexes in a number of ways (Razran, 1961). It is related to induction of the central state described as alertness or attention; it is not specific to the modality of stimulation employed and is initially generalized although, later, it may become restricted to a part of the body. Unlike other reaction patterns, those of the orienting reflex do not manage the initiating stimuli, but are merely reactive to their presence. Orienting reaction patterns are thus more preparatory than consummatory and are pre-adaptive rather than adaptive in nature. Futhermore, unlike specific reflexes, the orienting reflex tends to habituate rapidly upon stereotyped repetition of stimulation.

Indeed, the aspect of novelty seems to be the prepotent feature of stimuli evoking the orienting reflex (Sokolov, 1960). Its typical induction by non-stereotyped stimulation, has given rise to the concept that the orienting reflex is not initiated directly

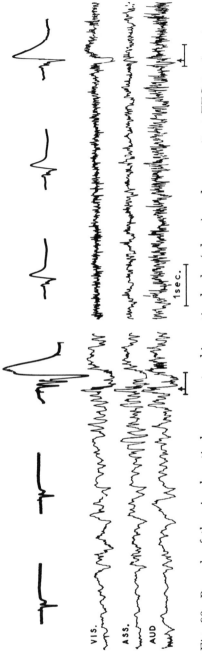

Fig. 60. Records of the visual cortical response to chiasmatic shocks (*above*) and concomitant EEG tracings in encéphale isolé. Note that facilitation of the visual response by reticular stimulation (signal below records) is much more pronounced during drowsiness (*left*), than during vigilance (*right*), and is most marked in the first 300 msec. of the arousing stimulus, corresponding to the Pavlovian orienting reflex. From Dumont and Dell (1960).

by the stimulus, in the customary sense of the term, but rather by a change in its intensity, temporal pattern or other parameter. A comparison of present with previous stimulation seems to be of major importance, with an orienting reflex being evoked at every point of disagreement. This reflex is induced whenever new stimuli are discordant, rather than accordant, with earlier stimulation.

The concept of a cortical neuronal model has been proposed by Sokolov (1960) to account for this induction of the orienting reflex by stimuli whose novelty is their characteristic feature. This neuronal model is conceived as a cortical cell assembly that preserves information about the modality, intensity, and duration and order of presentation of earlier stimuli, with which analagous aspects of novel stimulation may be compared (Fig. 61). According to the hypothesis, the orienting reflex is evoked whenever, upon such comparison, the parameters of the novel stimulus do not coincide with those of the neuronal model. This discordance,

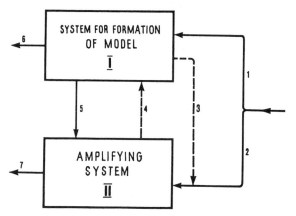

Fig. 61. Schema of the brain mechanisms involved in the orienting reflex. I. Cortical neuronal model; II. amplifying system in brain stem reticular formation. Functional connections are: 1. specific pathway from receptor to cortical neuronal model; 2. collateral afferent path to reticular formation; 3. negative feedback from cortical model to afferent reticular collateral; 4. ascending reticular activating pathway to cortex; 5. cortico-reticular connections signalling con- or dis-cordance between afferent stimuli and the cortical neuronal model; 6. corticifugal pathways for specific responses; 7. reticulofugal pathways for nonspecific somatic and visceral responses. From Sokolov (1960).

it is suggested, generates corticifugal discharge to the brain stem reticular system, the increased activity of which evokes the orienting reflex. In the contrasting situation, when novel stimuli are accordant with the proposed neuronal model, the cortex fails to excite the reticular system and the orienting reflex is not induced. Moreover, upon repetition, such accordance of stimulus and model is proposed to generate inhibitory corticifugal discharge to the brain stem, which blocks collateral afferent input to the reticular formation, and so promotes habituation.

While Sokolov's hypothesis acknowledges the participation of subcortical mechanisms in the orienting reflex, it proposes that they are managed and dominated by cortico-reticular influences. These, in turn, are generated by the comparison of novel stimuli with neuronal models established in the cortex by previous stimulation. Discordance between novel input and the model evokes excitatory cortico-reticular discharge, triggering the orienting reflex. Accordance of input and model fails to provoke the orienting reflex and, by promoting inhibitory cortico-reticular discharge, is responsible for habituation.

EXTERNAL INHIBITION

It was pointed out by Pavlov (1927) that, in the orienting reflex, the focus of attention upon an evocative signal blocks all extraneous stimulation and performance, by so-called external inhibition. "In our own laboratory," Pavlov wrote, "the neglect to provide against external stimuli often led to a curious complication when I visited some of my co-workers. Having by himself established a new conditioned reflex, working in the room with a dog, the experimenter would invite me for a demonstration and, then, everything would go wrong and he would be unable to show anything at all. It was I who presented this extra stimulus: the investigatory reflex was immediately brought into play; the dog gazed at me and smelled at me, and of course, this was sufficient to inhibit every recently established reflex."

Such external inhibition, associated with the orienting reflex, resembles the "sensory filtering" of Hernandez-Péon (1961) (see page 101),—managed by centrifugal reticular influences, reducing receptor sensitivity and transmission at lower sensory relays. It is to be differentiated from Pavlovian internal inhibition which, like habituation, appears to depend upon corticifugal inhibition of the reticular system. Pavlov (1927) pointed out that "the investigatory reflex invariably weakens on repetition and finally disappears altogether, in a manner resembling the extinction of conditioned reflexes." Further discussion of internal inhibition will be deferred to page 158.

REFERENCES

Adey, W. R., Segundo, J. P. and Livingston, R. B.: Corticofugal influences on intrinsic brain stem conduction in cat and monkey. *J. Neurophysiol.,* 20:1-16, 1957.

Bremer, F. and Terzuolo, C.: Nouvelles recherches sur le processus physiologique du réveil. *Arch. internat. Physiol.,* 61:86-90, 1953.

Dumont, S. and Dell, P.: Facilitation réticulaire des mécanismes visuels corticaux. *EEG Clin. Neurophysiol.,* 12:769-796, 1960.

Fangel, C. and Kaada, B. R.: Behavior "attention" and fear induced by cortical stimulation in the cat. *EEG Clin. Neurophysiol.,* 12:575-588, 1960.

Fernandez-Guardiola, A., Roldin, E., Fanjul, M. L. and Castells, C.: Role of the pupillary mechanism in the process of habituation of the visual pathways. *EEG Clin. Neurophysiol.,* 13:564-576, 1961.

French, J. D., Hernandez-Péon, R. and Livingston, R. B.: Projections from cortex to cephalic brain stem (reticular formation) in monkey. *J. Neurophysiol.,* 18:74-95, 1955.

Gardner, W. J., Licklider, J. C. R. and Weisz, A. Z.: Suppression of pain by sound. *Science, 132:*32-33, 1960.

Granit, R.: *Receptors and Sensory Perception.* New Haven, 1955.

Granit, R.: Centrifugal and antidromic effects on the ganglion cells of the retina. *J. Neurophysiol.,* 18:388-411, 1955.

Guzman Flores, C., Buendia, N., Anderson, C. and Lindsley, D. B.: Cortical and reticular influences upon evoked responses in dorsal column nuclei. *Exp. Neurol.,* 5:37-46, 1962.

Hagbarth, K. E. and Kerr, D. I. B.: Central influences on spinal afferent conduction. *J. Neurophysiol.,* 17:295-307, 1954.

Hernandez-Péon, R.: Central mechanisms controlling conduction along central sensory pathways. *Acta Neurol. Latinoamer., 1:*256-264, 1955.

Hernandez-Péon, R.: Neurophysiological correlates of habituation and other manifestations of plastic inhibition. In Jasper, H. H. and Smirnov, G. D. (Eds.) *Moscow Colloquium on EEG of Higher Nervous Activity. EEG Clin. Neurophysiol. Suppl., 13:*101-114, 1960.

Hernandez-Péon, R.: Reticular mechanisms of sensory control, pp. 497-520. In Rosenblith, W. (Ed.): *Sensory Communication*, M. I. T., Wiley, New York, 1961.

Hernandez-Péon, R., Scherrer, H. and Jouvet, M.: Modification of electrical activity in cochlear nucleus during "attention" in unanesthetized cats. *Science, 123*:331-332, 1956.

Hugelin, A. and Bonvallet, M.: Tonus corticale et contrôle de la facilitation motrice d'origine réticulaire. *J. Physiol., Paris, 49*:1171-1200, 1957.

Hugelin, A., Dumont, S. and Paillas, N.: Formation réticulaire et transmission des informations auditives au niveau de l'oreille moyenne et des voies acoustiques centrales. *EEG Clin. Neurophysiol., 12*:797-818, 1960.

Jasper, H. H., Ajmone-Marsan, C., and Stoll, J.: Corticofugal projections to the brain stem. *Arch. Neurol. & Psychiat., 67*:155-166, 1952.

John, E. R.: Higher Nervous Functions: Brain Functions and Learning. *Ann. Rev. Physiol., 23*:451-484, 1961.

Kaada, B. R. and Johannessen, N. B.: Generalized electrocortical activation by cortical stimulation in the cat. *EEG Clin. Neurophysiol., 12*:567-573, 1960.

Kuffler, S. W.: Neurons in the retina: organization, inhibition and excitation problems. *Cold Spring Harbor Symposia on Quant. Biology, 17*:281-292, 1952.

Kuypers, H. G. J. M.: Central cortical projections to motor and somatosensory cell groups. *Brain, 83*:161-184, 1960.

Lindblom, U. F. and Ottoson, J. O.: Effects of spinal sections on the spinal cord potentials elicited by stimulation of low-threshold cutaneous fibers. *Acta physiol. scandinav., 29*:Suppl. 106:191-208, 1953.

Mountcastle, V. B.: Some functional properties of the somatic afferent system, pp. 403-436. In Rosenblith, W. (Ed.) *Sensory Communication*. M. I. T. Wiley, New York, 1961.

Naquet, R., Regis, H., Fischer-Williams, M. and Fernandez-Guardiola, A.: Variations in the responses evoked by light along the specific pathways. *Brain, 83*:52-56, 1960.

Pavlov, I. P.: Conditioned reflexes; an investigation of the physiological activity of the cerebral cortex. Anrep, G. V. (Tr. and Ed.), Oxford Univ. Press, London, 1927.

Razran, G.: The observable unconscious and the inferable conscious in current Soviet psychophysiology: interoceptive conditioning, semantic conditioning and the orienting reflex. *Psychol. Rev., 68*:81-147, 1961.

Sharpless, S. and Jasper, H. H.: Habituation of the arousal reaction. *Brain, 79*:655-680, 1956.

Sokolov, E. N.: Neuronal models and the orienting reflex, pp. 187-276. In Brazier, M. A. B. (Ed.) *CNS and Behavior III*, Josiah Macy, Jr. Found., New York, 1960.

Solomon, P. (Ed.) *Sensory Deprivation.* Harvard Univ. Press, Cambridge, 1961.

Towe, A. L. and Jabbor, S. J.: Cortical inhibition of neurons in dorsal column nuclei of cat. *J. Neurophysiol., 24:*488-498, 1961.

Voronin, L. G. and Sokolov, E. N.: Cortical mechanisms of the orienting reflex and its relation to the conditioned reflex. In Jasper, H. H. and Smirnov, G. D. *Moscow Colloquium on EEG of Higher Nervous Activity. EEG Clin. Neurophysiol.* Suppl. *13:*335-346, 1960.

7

CONTRIBUTIONS TO THE
ELECTROPHYSIOLOGY OF LEARNING

Much recent progress in the study of higher nervous activity has come from electrophysiological analysis of the mechanisms of learned behavior. Knowledge has especially been advanced by a marriage between the electrical recording techniques of Western neurophysiology and the classical Pavlovian approaches to study of conditional reflexes, cultivated so extensively in the USSR (Jasper and Smirnov, 1960; Delafresnaye, 1960; Brazier, 1959, 1960; Kline, 1961). While pioneering studies of the electrical activity of the brain during learning were undertaken in the USSR in the nineteen thirties and more recently have been extended by a considerable number of Soviet investigators, reviewed by Rusinov and Rabinovich (1958), these findings are just now becoming available in English translation and Western knowledge of them is still regrettably limited.

ELECTROCORTICAL CONDITIONING

Western work in this field similarly began in the thirties when Durup and Fessard (1935), in study of the alpha-blocking response to visual stimulation, noted that an associated click of their camera soon itself elicited alpha-blocking, even when the visual stimulus was not presented. This adventitious finding was confirmed and extended by Jasper and Shagass (1941) and more recently, the method has been employed by Morrell and his associates (1953, 1956, 1957, 1958, 1959, 1961), as a means of studying the formation of temporary connections in the brain during simulated conditioning procedures. Such "learned" blocking of the alpha rhythm is illustrated in Figure 62 (Morrell and Ross, 1953). An initial lack of cortical response to a tone, in A, contrasts with the unconditional blocking of the occipital alpha

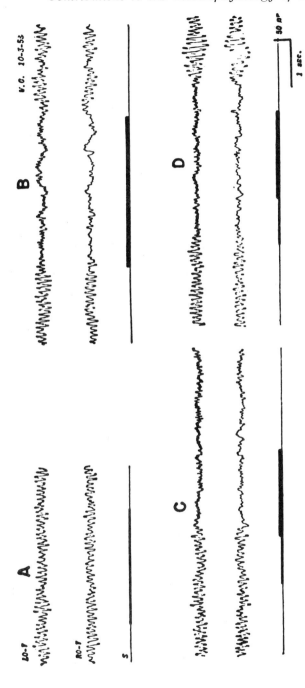

Fig. 62. Records of electrical activity from the brain of a normal human subject, illustrating the establishment of a conditional blocking of occipital alpha rhythm. The initial lack of response to a tone stimulus (thin black signal) is seen in A. The unconditioned alpha blockade to bright light stimulation (thick black signal) is seen in B. When the signals are first paired (C), the tone stimulus preceding the light is ineffective. By the ninth trial, in D, however, the tone stimulus evokes a conditional alpha-blocking response before the light appears. From Morrell and Ross (1953).

rhythm, induced by a bright light stimulus, in B. In the first paired trial (C), the lack of response to the tone again contrasts with alpha blocking when the light appears. By the ninth trial, in D, however, alpha blocking occurs in response to the tone, before the light is presented. At this initial stage, conditional alpha blocking is displayed widely over the cortex; subsequently, it becomes confined to the occipital region, that is, to the projection area of the unconditional signal.

These observations indicate that, by appropriate association and repetition of two signals, a previously indifferent conditional stimulus can ultimately evoke the EEG arousal response induced initially only by unconditional stimulation. As Pavlov (Koshtoyants, 1955) proposed, novel functional connections must be established to subserve such learned behavior. Appropriately, these records of conditioned changes in electrical activity were obtained from the cerebral cortex which, according to Pavlov, is the preeminent site of formation of such novel, adaptive, temporary, conditional, neural links. Furthermore, the consecutive alterations of electrocortical events, at first widespread and subsequently focal, appear to parallel the succession of initial generalization and later differentiation, identified by Pavlov in the establishment of every conditional reflex. Additionally, the observation that recordable alterations are most conspicuous in the cortical analyzer, or receiving area, for the unconditional signal, suggests the possibility that this site may be the dominant focus of the change.

In a later variation of electrocortical conditioning, Morrell and Jasper (1956) employed intermittent, rather than steady photic stimulation as the unconditional signal. At a stage between the initial general and the final focal desynchronization of the EEG, they observed in the visual cortex, again in the focus of the unconditioned analyzer, a tone-induced, repetitive response, the frequency of which was that of photic stimulation. In extension of these experiments Yoshii *et al.* (1957) found that the conditioned repetitive discharge was earlier in onset, higher in amplitude and more constant in subcortical structures, especially in the mesencephalic reticular formation (Fig. 63). In subsequent study, Yoshii and Hockaday (1958), found this conditional frequency specific response to be prevented by bilateral lesions in non-specific thalamic nuclei. Lesions of the diencephalon and midbrain have similarly been reported to interfere with conditioning by Doty (1959); and Morrell (1961) has likewise supported the involvement of non-specific mechanisms of the brain stem in electrocortical conditioning.

In similar fashion, it has been proposed by Gastaut (1958) that closure in conditional learning is not completed within the cortex, for interruptions of connections between the cortical analyzers, or removal of one of them, does not prevent closure. Alternatively, Gastaut proposes that linkage is established at the sites of convergence of signals within the reticular formation or midline thalamic nuclei of the brain stem. As seen in Figure 64,

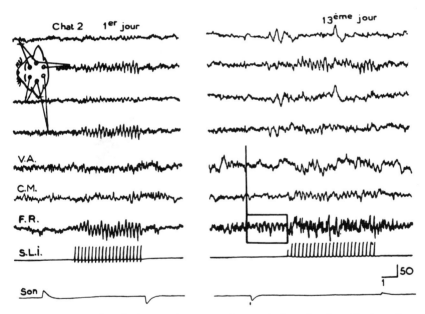

Fig. 63. Records of electrical activity in cortical and subcortical regions of the cat's brain, showing responses to tone (TON) and intermittent photic (SLI) stimulation. On the first day (*left*), the sound is without effect, and one observes only the unconditioned driving of the occipital and reticular activity at the frequency of the light flashes. On the thirteenth day (*right*), the sound evoked a conditional response at the same frequency as the rhythmic light flashes, recorded only from the reticular formation. From Yoshii, Pruvot and Gastaut (1957).

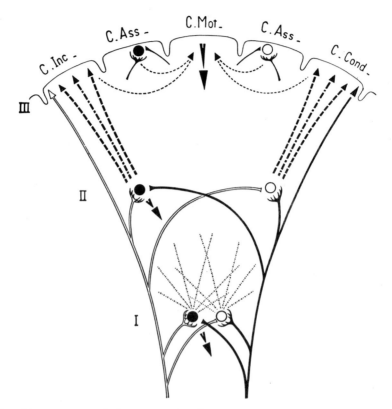

Fig. 64. Diagram of the proposed subcortical and cortical levels involved in coupling between stimuli in the establishment of conditioned learning. I. Reticular formation of lower brain stem. II. Thalamic reticular formation. III. Cerebral cortex. From Gastaut (1958).

he conceives of the setting up of a reticular focus of excitation, by way of collaterals from the afferent paths for the unconditioned stimulus, with the establishment of connections between it and the cortex; and with the subsequent domination of localized thalamo-cortical projections over more diffuse ones from lower levels, as the ultimate changes become focal rather than generalized. Paradoxically, these developments of Western neurophysiology, initially concerned with study of electrocortical changes in learning, have thus come to emphasize the importance of convergence of signals in the central brain stem, in proposing a subcortical rather than a cortical genesis of the learning process.

INFLUENCE OF REINFORCEMENT IN LEARNING

Further Western emphasis upon the importance of subcortical mechanisms in learning, has come from study of brain stem mechanisms for the orienting reflex and attention, with which all learning begins (discussed on pages 109-112), and of the role in learning of reinforcement, the limbic mechanisms for which are at the very core of the unconditional reflex (discussed on pages 59-63). Valuable progress has been made by monitoring tracer responses, evoked in central neural stations by afferent stimulation, before and during reinforcement procedures. In the experiments of John and Killam (1959) novel photic stimuli, which initially evoked widespread central activity, were repeatedly presented until their amplitude and distribution became confined to the visual pathway in habituation (Fig. 65, above). Immediately thereafter, when negative reinforcement was introduced, by pairing shocks to the feet with the tracer stimuli, central responses again became widely generalized and displayed a marked increase in amplitude (Fig. 65, below). In similar experiments of Galambos (1959) and of Hearst *et al.* (1960), tone-evoked responses in the hippocampus were conspicuously augmented when positive reinforcement was introduced (Fig. 66). These recent findings along with those of Jouvet and Hernandez-Péon *et al.* (1957) and of Worden (1959), demonstrate the important role of reinforcement in augmenting the amplitude and increasing the distribution of afferent signals through the brain.

Significantly, these changes in tracer responses during training similarly followed the pattern of initial generalization and subsequent differentiation, identified generally in the formation of a conditional reflex. The widespread distribution of responses early in reinforcement became much more restricted as learned behavior was established and, ultimately, evoked potentials were limited to the cortical area for the unconditioned signal. From these observations, it would no longer seem necessary, in accounting for the establishment of temporary connections, to search for limited sites of convergence between isolated signals. Moreover, the average response analysis of Brazier (1961) has

HABITUATION

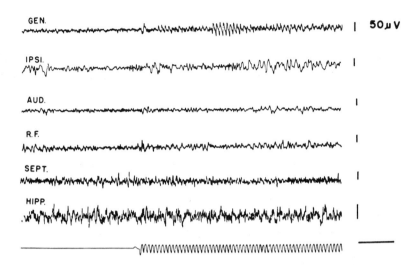

1ST DAY OF TRAINING

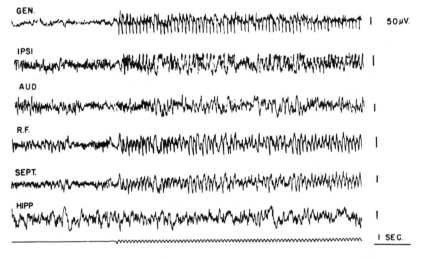

Fig. 65. Records of electrical activity from cortical and subcortical regions of the cat's brain, showing (*above*) the minimal and restricted response to repetitive photic stimulation (signal) after habituation; and (*below*) the marked increase in amplitude and the widespread generalization of responses when reinforcement is introduced. From John and Killam (1959).

shown that, even without reinforcement, afferent potentials evoked in unanesthetized animals are much more widely distributed in the brain than previous concepts of modality segregation have allowed. From such recent studies, the problem would seem rather to lie in determining in which of many possible sites, new functional relationships may become preserved.

The functions of analysis, discrimination and differentiation involve aspects of neural performance implicit in the concept developed by Pavlov (Koshtoyants, 1955) of a dominant focus in learning, conceived as a central core of excitation with an inhibitory surround (see page 105). The active role of inhibition in differentiation relates to the importance of what has since been called the falling out of components in the learning

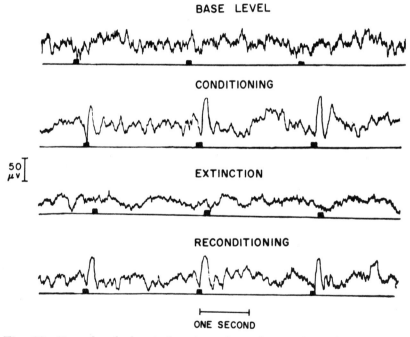

Fig. 66. Records of electrical activity from the monkey's hippocampus, showing (from above downward) variations in the responses evoked by tone stimuli: during the control period; during reinforcement with sugar pellets in conditioning; after extinction; and during subsequent reconditioning (with food reward again presented). From Hearst, Beer, Sheatz, and Galambos (1960).

process. Recent knowledge of the inhibitory cortico-reticular and sensory control mechanisms of the brain may be of relevance here (see pages 100-106).

PHYSIOLOGICAL ARCHITECTURE OF THE CONDITIONAL REFLEX

In a new conception of the physiological architecture of the conditional reflex, Anokhin (1961) has identified four sequential steps, illustrated in Figure 67. They consist: first, of a stage of *afferent synthesis,* to which both specific and nonspecific inputs contribute; second, a stage of elaboration of an *acceptor of action,* conceived as a complex of excitation formed in the cortex by previous experience; third, a stage of *formation of the effector apparatus;* and fourth, a stage of *return afferentation.* Of this last, Anokhin (1961) remarks "The conception of 'return afferentation' had developed in our laboratory long before the cybernetic trend of thinking led to the formulation of the 'feedback' idea, now being transferred into neurophysiology and proposed for self-regulatory, technical systems."

Anokhin's concept, which in some degree resembles that of Sokolov (1960) (see pages 111-112), emphasizes that "It is precisely at the point where the excitation of the acceptor of action, and the stream of return afferentations from the results of the action, meet, that the necessary condition for coordinated and regulated relation of the animal and man to the external environment lies. Only when these two streams of excitation coincide exactly, do the effector excitations cease to reach the functioning apparatus and is the given behavior stage in the chain of individual reflex actions completed." More generally, Anokhin continues "If the streams of return afferentations, entering the brain along different analyzers, fail to coincide with the systems of

———————————————————————————————————→

Fig. 67. Physiological architecture of conditioned reflex, showing: I. stage of afferent synthesis (A-analyzer system; a-reticular system); II. stage of formation of acceptor of action; III. stage of formation of effector apparatus; and IV. stage of return afferentation of the results of conditioned reflex action. From Anokhin (1961).

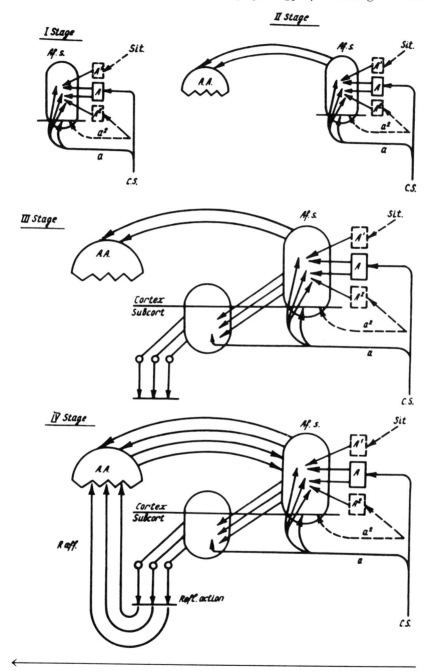

excitation, which has formed at the end of the afferent synthesis, and is the opposite of the acceptor of action, this lack of coincidence immediately involves other reactions, primarily the orienting-investigatory reflex. In any act of behavior, this cyclic process, beginning with the afferent synthesis stage and ending in the confrontation of the return afferentations and the excitations of the acceptor of action, continues until both excitations fully coincide." It is of great interest that both the Pavlovian orienting reflex and the Pavlovian conditional reflex have recently received conceptual interpretation by Soviet neurophysiologists in cybernetical terms.

REFERENCES

Anokhin, P. K.: A new conception of the physiological architecture of conditioned reflex. Pp. 189-229. In Delafresnaye, J. F. (Ed.) *Brain Mechanisms and Learning*. Blackwell, Oxford, 1961.

Brazier, M. A. B. (Ed.): *CNS and Behavior*. Trans. first, second and third Macy Conferences. Josiah Macy, Jr. Foundation, New York, 1959 (a and b), 1960.

Brazier, M. A. B.: Paired sensory modality stimulation studied by computer analysis. Pp. 1054-1063. In Kline, N. S.: *Pavlovian Conference on Higher Nervous Activity*. Ann. N.Y. Acad. Sci., 92:1054-1063, 1961.

Delafresnaye, J. F. (Ed.): *Brain Mechanisms and Learning*. Blackwell, Oxford, 1961.

Doty, R. W.: Brain stimulation and conditioned reflexes. Pp. 241-306. Brazier, M. A. B. (Ed.) *CNS and Behavior*. Josiah Macy, Jr. Foundation, New York, 1959.

Durup, G. and Fessard, A.: L'électroencéphalogramme de l'homme; observations psycho-physiologiques rélatives à l'action des stimuli visuals et auditifs. *Année Psychol.*, 36:1-32, 1935.

Galambos, R.: Electrical correlates of learning. Pp. 375-415. In Brazier, M. A. B. (Ed.): *CNS and Behavior*, Josiah Macy, Jr. Foundation, New York, 1959.

Gastaut, H.: État actuel des connaissances sur l'électroencéphalographie du conditionnement. *EEG Clin. Neurophysiol. Suppl.*, 6:133, 1957.

Gastaut, H.: Some aspects of the neurophysiological basis of conditioned reflexes and behavior. Pp. 255-276. In Wolstenholme, G. E. W. and O'Connor, C. M. (Eds.) *Neurological Basis of Behavior*, Little Brown, Boston, 1958.

Gastaut, H.: The role of the reticular formation in establishing conditioned reactions. Pp. 561-589. In Jasper, H. H. (Ed.) *Reticular Formation of the Brain*, Little Brown, Boston, 1958.

Hearst, E., Beer, B., Sheatz, G. and Galambos, R.: Some electrophysiological correlates of conditioning in the monkey. *EEG Clin. Neurophysiol.*, 12:137-152, 1960.

Hernandez-Péon, R., Scherer, H. and Jouvet, M.: Modification of electrical activity in cochlear nucleus during "attention" in unanesthetized cats. *Science, 123:*331-332, 1956.

Jasper, H. H. and Shagass, C.: Conditioning the occipital alpha rhythm in man. *J. Exp. Psychol.*, 28:373-388, 1941.

Jasper, H. H. and Smirnov, G. D. (Eds.): *Moscow Colloquium on Electroencephalography of Higher Nervous Activity. EEG Clin. Neurophysiol. Suppl. 13*, 1960.

John, E. R.: Higher nervous functions: brain functions and learning. *Ann. Rev. Physiol.*, 23:451-484, 1961.

John, E. R. and Killam, K. F.: Electrophysiological correlates of avoidance conditioning in the cat. *J. Pharm. Exper. Therap.*, 125:252-274, 1959.

Jouvet, M. and Hernandez-Péon, R.: Mechanismes neurophysiologiques concernant l'habituation, l'attention et le conditionement. *EEG Clin. Neurophysiol. Suppl.*, 6:39-49, 1957.

Koshtoyants, K. S. (Ed.): *I. P. Pavlov, Selected Works.* Foreign Lang. Publ. House, Moscow, 1955.

Magoun, H. W.: Subcortical mechanisms for reinforcement. Jasper, H. H. and Smirnov, G. D. (Eds.) *Moscow Colloquium on Electroencephalography of Higher Nervous Activity. EEG Clin. Neurophysiol. Suppl.*, 13:221-229, 1960.

Magoun, H. W.: Recent contributions to the electrophysiology of learning. In Kline, N. S. (Ed.) *Pavlovian Conference on Higher Nervous Activity. Ann. N.Y. Acad. Sci.*, 92:818-829, 1961.

Morrell, F. and Ross, M.: Central inhibition in cortical conditioned reflexes. *AMA Arch. Neurol. & Psychiat.*, 70:611-616, 1953.

Morrell, F. and Jasper, H. H.: Electrographic studies of the formation of temporary connections of the brain. *EEG Clin. Neurophysiol.*, 8:201-215, 1956.

Morrell, F., Naquet, R. and Gastaut, H.: Evolution of some electrical signs of conditioning: 1. Normal cat and rabbit. *J. Neurophysiol.*, 20:574-587, 1957.

Morrell, F.: Some electrical events involved in the formation of temporary connections. Pp. 545-560. In Jasper, H. H. (Ed.) *Reticular Formation of the Brain.* Little Brown, Boston, 1958.

Morrell, F.: Electroencephalographic studies of conditioned learning. Pp. 307-374. In Brazier, M. A. B. (Ed.) *CNS and Behavior.* Josiah Macy, Jr., Foundation, New York, 1959.

Morrell, F.: Electrophysiological contributions to the neural basis of learning. *Physiol. Rev.*, 41:443-494, 1961.

Pavlov, I. P.: *Scientific Session on the Physiological Teachings of Academician I. P. Pavlov.* Foreign Lang. Pub. House, Moscow, 1951.

Razran, G.: A Survey of experiments in interoceptive conditioning, semantic conditioning and orienting reflex. *Psych. Rev., 68*:81-147, 1961.

Rusinov, V. S. and Rabinovich, M. Y.: Electroencephalographic researches in the laboratories and clinics of the Soviet Union. *EEG Clin. Neurophysiol. Suppl. 8, 1-36,* 1958.

Sokolov, E. N.: Neuronal models and the orienting influence, pp. 187-276. In Brazier, M. A. B.: *CNS and Behavior.* Josiah Macy, Jr. Foundation, New York, 1960.

Voronin, L. G. and Sokolov, E. N.: Cortical mechanisms of the orienting reflex and its relation to the conditioned reflex. In Jasper, H. H. and Smirnov, G. D. (Eds.) *Electroencephalography of Higher Nervous Activity. EEG Clin. Neurophysiol. Suppl., 13*:335-346, 1960.

Worden, F. G.: Neurophysiological contributions to the understanding of schizophrenia. In Auerbach, E. (Ed.) *Schizophrenia, An Integrated Approach.* Ronald Press, New York, 1959.

Yoshii, N.: Principes methodologiques de l'investigation électroéncephalogique du comportement conditionne. *EEG Clin. Neurophysiol. Suppl., 6*:75-88, 1957.

Yoshii, N., Pruvot, P. and Gastaut, H.: Electroencephalographic activity of the mesencephalic reticular formation during conditioning in the cat. *EEG Clin. Neurophysiol., 9*:595-608, 1957.

Yoshii, N. and Hockaday, W. J.: Conditioning of frequency-characteristic repetitive EEG response with intermittent photic stimulation. *EEG Clin. Neurophysiol., 10*:487-502, 1958.

8

PROCESSING OF INFORMATION INTO MEMORY

IT IS REMARKABLE how recurringly man has sought an understanding of the memory process in terms of the formation of a physical trace or imprint upon some component of the brain. In Plato's *Dialogues* (Jowett, 1931), Socrates proposed that "There exists in the mind of man a block of wax—of different sizes and qualities in different men. This tablet is a gift of Memory, the mother of the Muses; and when we wish to remember anything—which we have seen or heard or thought—we hold the wax to it and, in that material, receive its impression as from the seal of a ring. We remember and know what is imprinted as long as the image lasts, but when it is effaced or cannot be taken, then we forget and do not know."

There is much recent indication that components of the temporal region of the brain, in particular the hippocampus and entorhinal cortex, serve importantly in processing novel information into storage, as well as in its early consolidation and recall. The role of this region in memory function was first proposed by gifted clinical investigators concerned with the involvement of this part of the brain in disease.

TEMPORAL LOBE SEIZURES

Attention to changes in memory in temporal lobe seizures began with Hughlings Jackson's (1888) report of the case of Z. The patient was himself a highly educated physician, with recurring attacks which invariably began with an aura of intense recollection—of what he did not know, for the succeeding seizure, spreading through the temporal lobe, from an uncinate focus observed at autopsy (Fig. 68), paralyzed function and prevented both processing of the experience into memory and its subsequent recall. In more recent observations, Feindel and

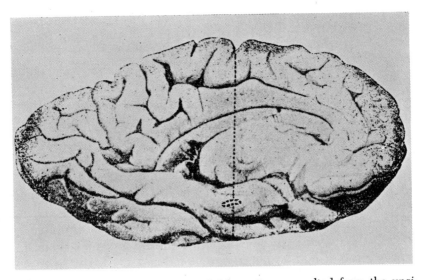

Fig. 68. Brain of Z, whose temporal lobe seizures resulted from the uncinate focus found at autopsy (from Hughlings Jackson, 1888).

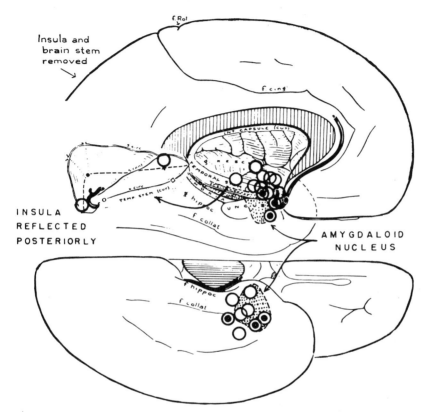

Fig. 69. Medial and inferior aspects of the hemisphere of man, with circles marking the points at which stimulation produced after-discharge and automatism. From Feindel and Penfield (1954).

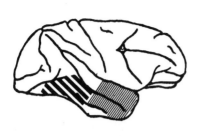
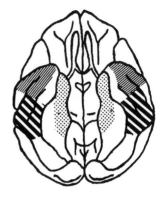

 Superior Temporal Ablations

Inferior Temporal Ablations

Amygdalo-hippocampal complex Ablations

Fig. 70. Lateral and ventral views of monkey's brain, showing the distribution of experimental lesions of the temporal lobe. Hippocampal lesions (stipple) resulted in memory defect. From Stepien, Cordeau and Rasmussen (1960).

Penfield (1954) have found it possible, by direct electrical stimulation of the hippocampus (Fig. 69), to trigger such temporal lobe seizures, characterized both by auras of recollection, or *déja vu*, as well as by interruption of memory processing and retrograde amnesia. In his wide neurosurgical experience, Penfield (1959) has found the lateral temporal cortex to be the only brain region from which actual earlier remembered experience can be reinvoked or triggered by direct stimulation and this only in patients with seizures and probable alteration of function of this part of the brain.

KORSAKOFF'S SYNDROME

A second line of clinical evidence for hippocampal involvement in memory function was initiated by Korsakoff (1890), whose classic description of the psychosis bearing his name, emphasized the paradoxically severe impairment of recent memory, along with the preservation of that for earlier periods (Talland, 1960). In his cases of alcoholic neuritis or senile atrophy, pathology was widespread in the brain. A number of subsequent cases have been reported, however, in which focal, bilateral destruction of the hippocampus was observed at autopsy in cases of classical Korsakoff's syndrome (Victor *et al.*, 1961).

Still more definite reference has come from recent neurosurgical ablation of the temporal lobes for the relief of psychomotor seizures (Scoville, 1954; Penfield and Milner, 1958; Milner, 1958). These surgical patients presented syndromes like those of Korsakoff's patients; they were incapable of processing current experience into memory and impairment of recall extended backward, with diminishing severity, for as long as two to four years before operation. Earlier memories could still be recollected vividly, however. While the ablated neural region must serve importantly in the processing of memory, as well as in its early fixation and retrieval, it obviously cannot be considered to provide the storehouse for all memories once induced. Such storage must be served by other portions of the brain and doubtless involves widespread cerebral participation.

EXPERIMENTAL TEMPORAL LOBECTOMY

These clinical observations have been supported by animal studies in which bilateral ablations of the temporal lobes and, more particularly, the hippocampus, have resulted in severe memory defects, inferred from behavior or tested in learning situations. Following early bilateral temporal lobectomy in the monkey, Brown and Schäffer (1888) may be said to have prematurely discovered the Klüver-Bucy syndrome (1939). Their animals exhibited the same perseverative handling or mouthing of familiar objects, as though they were novel, and displayed the same symptoms described later as visual agnosia, which seemingly are primarily manifestations of memory impairment.

More recent work of Stepien, Rasmussen and their associates (1960), as well as Orbach *et al.* (1960), Kaada *et al.* (1961), and others has shown that both in the rat and monkey, hippocampal ablation (Fig. 70) is the significant lesion and a resultant

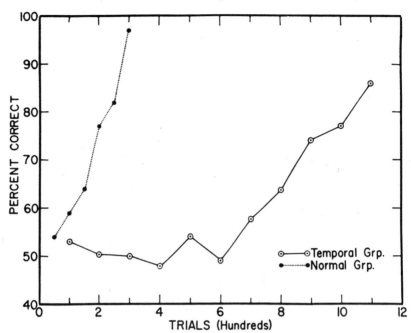

Fig. 71. Learning curves on visual pattern discrimination task, in control monkeys (*upper left*), and monkeys with seizures following alumina cream lesions of the inferior temporal region (*lower right*). From Stamm and Pribram (1961).

memory defect, rather than a visual or emotional disturbance, is the significant factor, responsible for impaired acquisition of discriminative performance or avoidance learning in such preparations, although previously learned tasks may be retained. In the experiments of Stamm and Pribram (1961), recurring seizures induced in the monkey by alumina cream lesions of the temporal lobe, greatly retarded and reduced the acquisition of learned behavior (Fig. 71). The effect upon avoidance learning of reversible, bilateral, hippocampal, spreading depression has been observed by Bureš (1959) in the rat. Conditioned reflexes were almost completely abolished and "it was as if there were a complete memory loss of what had occurred immediately before." These many observations seem clearly to implicate the hippocampus, and probably the adjacent entorhinal temporal cortex, in the induction and consolidation of memory, as well as in its early recall; though other portions of the brain must just as clearly constitute the ultimate storehouse of remembered experience (Deutsch, 1962).

HIPPOCAMPAL THETA RHYTHM

Obviously, to serve in memory processing, the hippocampus must be activated by the whole spectrum of experiential input to the brain. In addition to forward passage in classical sensory paths, all afferent signals evoke ascending activity in less specific routes through the central brain stem and medial diencephalon (see pages 81-85). This central transmission continues farther to the septum and is conducted into the hippocampus by centripetal fibers of the fornix (Green and Adey, 1956; Petsche *et al.*, 1962).

A severe impairment of learning when the activity of the central cephalic brain stem is jammed by direct electrical stimulation (Mahut, 1957; Ingram, 1958; Thompson, 1958; Olds and Olds, 1961), or blocked with lesions (King, 1958; Doty *et al.*, 1959; Hernandez-Péon and Brust-Carmona, 1961) may depend essentially upon interruption of afferent signals to the hippocampus. The fixation and recall of memory are similarly vulnerable to electro-shock, drugs and, in man, cerebral concussion (Gerard, 1955). Reference has been made earlier (page 69) to the possible role of external inhibition, associated with release of the orienting reflex, after frontal or temporal lobectomy, in blocking impulse traffic to and from the hippocampal system, and so contributing to the memory impairment associated with the excessive distractibility of such preparations.

On reaching the hippocampus, all input seems equivalently capable of evoking a ubiquitous pattern of electrical activity called the theta rhythm (Fig. 72); first observed by Jung and Kornmuller (1938), and since contributed to importantly by Liberson and Cadhilac (1953), and by Green, Adey and their associates and others. As seen in Figure 73, from Green and Arduini (1954), the theta rhythm consists of regularly recurring, large amplitude, slow waves at a frequency of 4-7 per second, which form as characteristic a pattern of hippocampal activation as does the contrasting low-voltage, fast pattern of neocortical

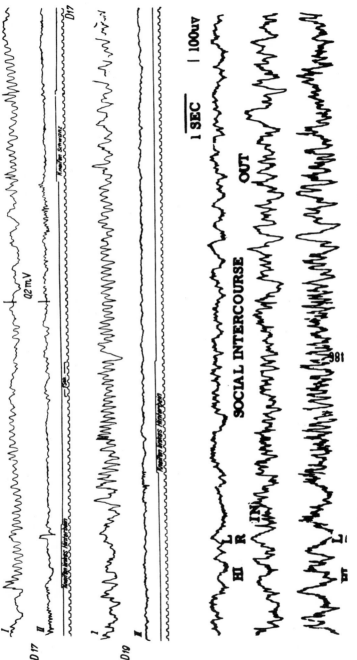

Fig. 72. Early records of hippocampal theta activity, induced (*above*) in rabbit by pinching leg and tail, with control records from caudate nucleus. From Jung and Kornmüller (1938). Theta rhythm, induced (*below*) in guinea pig by experimenter entering room and talking to animal, with control record from neocortex. From Liberson and Cadhilac (1953).

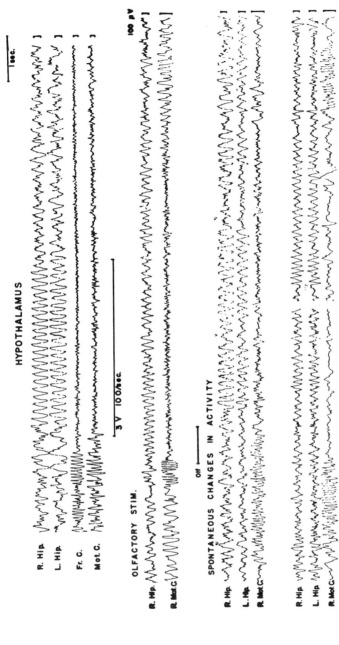

Fig. 73. Records of electrical activity of hippocampus (Hip) and neocortex (Fr and Mot) of rabbit, showing theta rhythms evoked by hypothalamic (*above*), and olfactory (*middle*) stimulation, and appearing spontaneously (*below*), in each instance concomitantly with low fast pattern in neocortical EEG. From Green and Arduini (1954).

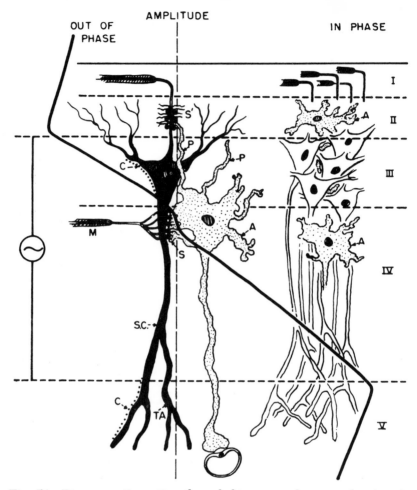

Fig. 74. Diagrammatic section through hippocampal cortex, showing the relations of pyramidal cells and astrocytes. As determined by microelectrode recording, the amplitude of the plotted theta wave (*heavy line*) passes through zero potential, i.e., turns over, in the region of the proximal portion of the apical dendrite. From Green (1959).

EEG-arousal, of which the theta rhythm is invariably a concomitant.

On the basis of their studies in the rabbit, Green (1959) and Green *et al.* (1960) conclude that the theta rhythm arises from longitudinal currents flowing between the soma of the hippocampal pyramidal cells and the proximal portion of their apical dendrites (Fig. 74). The waves themselves represent graded, non-propagated, electrotonic changes, from varying phases of which arise the propagating, pulse-coded, digital output responsible for transfer of information to other parts of the brain.

A current program of Adey (1961) and Adey *et al.* (1958, 1960 a and b) is exploring changes in the hippocampal theta rhythm during approach learning in the cat. In the naïve animal (Fig. 75, above), the conditional signal evokes irregularly-ranging theta frequencies, distributed widely in the hippocampal region. With development of a learned response, however (Fig. 75, below), the theta pattern becomes restricted in its major representation to the dorsal hippocampus and entorhinal cortex, and its amplitude and frequency-spectrum become conspicuously regular and invariable. In extension of this work, Adey *et al.* (1960, 1961) have employed computer methods to study phase relationships between theta patterns in the hippocampus proper and those in the adjacent entorhinal temporal cortex during stages of approach learning. As seen in Figure 76 (left), during early stages of acquisition of learned behavior, when it may be inferred that information is being processed into memory, theta waves in the hippocampus lead those in the adjacent temporal lobe, suggesting impulse traffic from hippocampus to cortex. By contrast in the well-trained animal (Fig. 76, right), when one may infer that the conditional signal evokes recall, entorhinal theta waves lead those in the hippocampus, suggesting impulse traffic in the inverse direction, from cortex into hippocampus.

In physical systems, the match of variable signals against some type of yardstick has been shown to possess advantages for information-processing beyond those afforded by the capacities of a single channel operating by itself alone. Rather than itself conveying information, the highly stabilized theta rhythm can be suggested to serve as a phase-comparator or carrier wave (Adey *et al.*, 1960, 1961), or a scale or comparison generator (Brazier, 1960), against which more variably patterned, information-conveying signals, arriving concomitantly over other channels, can be compared or measured, with the combination of the two leading to the establishment of traces wherever memories are stored.

Adey (1961) has conceived that these shifting patterns of wave discharge, which display characteristic alterations with stages of the learning process, may serve causally in the induction of enduring biochemical modifications in the neurons affected or involved. Previous proposals along this line have usually emphasized changes at the surface of the nerve cell, particularly those induced at synaptic terminals by short-lasting nerve impulses. By contrast, Adey (1961) has stressed the probable importance of alterations within the sub-surface, intra-cellular cytoplasm of the post-synaptic neuron, consequent upon much more prolonged changes in membrane polarization—and the duration of a theta wave is of the order of 200 ms.; or of more prolonged changes still, involving intermediate or associated participation of neuroglia.

NEUROGLIAL FUNCTION

Neurophysiologists are at last beginning to devote attention to the functions of neuroglia, which collectively form about half the bulk and some nine-tenths of the cells making up the brain. On impaling a glial cell in tissue culture with a micro-electrode, Hild and Tasaki (1962), have recorded a resting potential equivalent to that of a neuron (Fig. 77, upper trace) and, with stimulus-pulses, have induced transient reductions of glial membrane polarization, which return to normal over a period of about five seconds. Similar non-propagating alterations have been recorded (Fig. 77, lower trace) from what are assumed to be glial cells in the cat's cerebral cortex.

In micro-electrode studies of the fish retina, Svaetichin and his associates (1961) have impaled glial components and recorded potential alterations, induced by photic stimulation (Fig. 78), the latencies of which are about 50 ms., the peaks about 500 ms., and the total duration more than a second long. As Gliambos (1961) has recently pointed out, glial cells certainly are able to respond to stimulation and display capacities for continued alteration of function, far longer than those customarily associated with neuronal discharge.

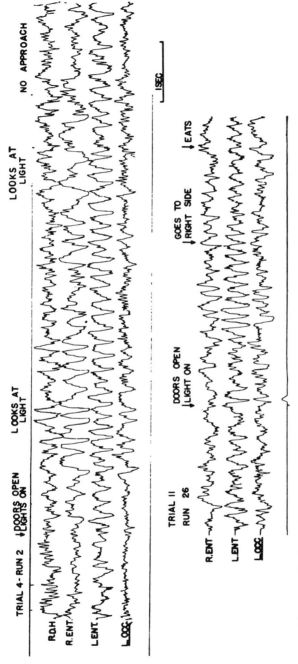

Fig. 75. Records from hippocampus (RDH), entorhinal (ENT) and occipital (OCC) cortex of cat, showing differing patterns of theta rhythm, during early trial (*above*) and after acquisition of approach learning (*below*). From Adey (1961).

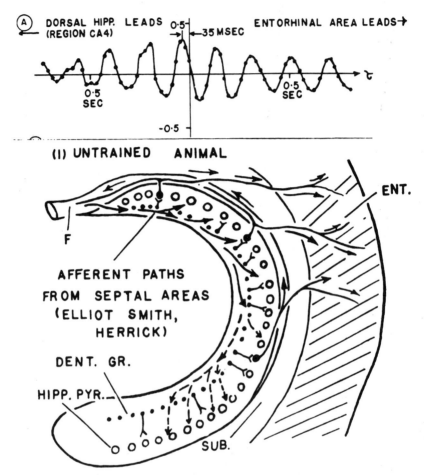

Fig. 76. Cross correlations between dorsal hippocampal and entorhinal records of theta rhythm, in early training stage of approach learning (*left*), and in the fully trained cat (*right*). In the untrained animal, the hippocampal waves lead those in the entorhinal area, suggesting a sequence of activity from hippocampus to cortex (*left*). In the trained animal, the entorhinal waves now lead those in the hippocampus, suggesting a contrasting sequence of activity from cortex to hippocampus (*right*). From Adey, Dunlop and Hendrix (1960) and Adey, Walter and Hendrix (1961).

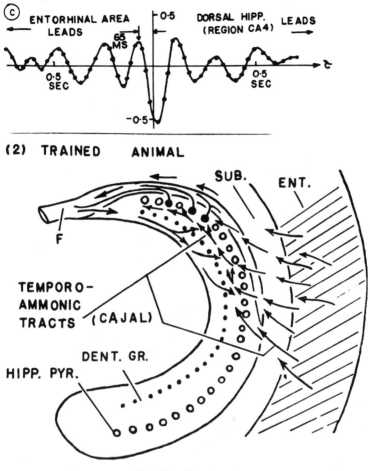

Fig. 76—*Continued*

ELECTRON MICROSCOPY OF GLIAL-NEURONAL RELATIONS

Current electron microscopic studies by Pease and his associates (1957) and others, have stressed the intimate structural association of glial and neuronal elements in the brain. Their photographs (Fig. 79) show the astrocytic glial, transport system surrounding capillaries (right), cut transversely (above) and longitudinally (below). Other processes of the same astro-

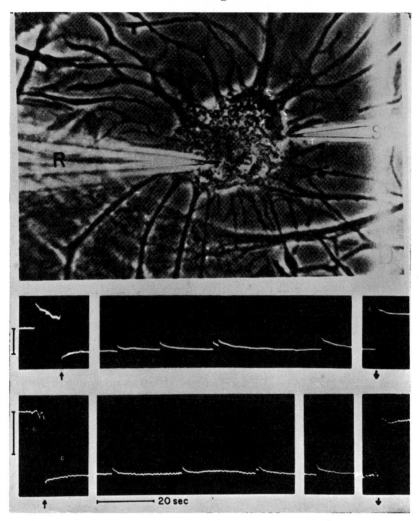

Fig. 77. Photomicrograph (*above*) of living kitten astrocyte in tissue culture, impaled by a recording microelectrode (R), with a stimulating electrode (S) at right. Upper record shows resting potential of glial cell membrane, on penetrating and withdrawing from cell (*arrows*), and prolonged depolarization induced by repeated stimulation (*center*). Lower record shows similar resting potential and responses from a "glial" element in cat cortex. Calibration mV (*above*) and 50 mV (*below*). From Hild and Tasaki (1962).

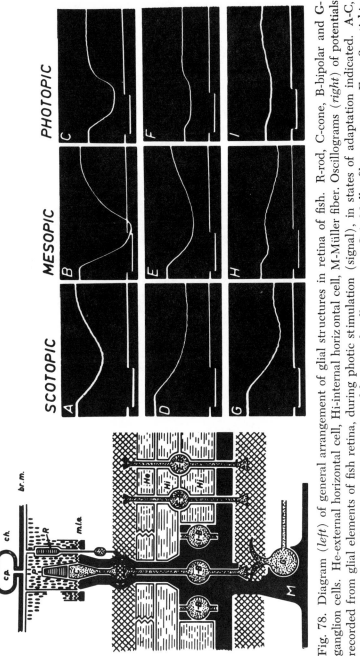

Fig. 78. Diagram (*left*) of general arrangement of glial structures in retina of fish. R-rod, C-cone, B-bipolar and G-ganglion cells. He-external horizontal cell, Hi-internal horizontal cell, M-Müller fiber. Oscillograms (*right*) of potentials recorded from glial elements of fish retina, during photic stimulation (signal), in states of adaptation indicated. A-C, external horizontal cell responses; D-F, internal horizontal cell responses; G-1, Müller fiber responses. From Svaetichin *et al.* (1961) and Mitarai *et al.* (1961).

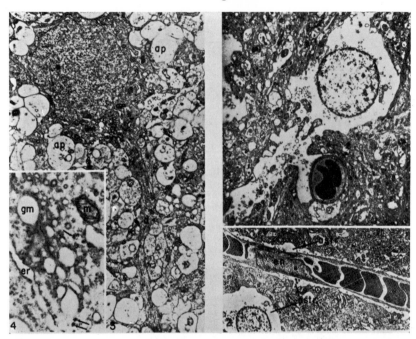

Fig. 79. Electron micrographs from rat cerebral cortex showing cell body of astrocyte (*upper right*), processes of which surround transversely (*above*) and longitudinally (*below*) sectioned capillaries. At left, other branches of astrocytic processes (ap) make abundant contact with soma and dendrite of small neuron. From Maynard *et al.* (1957) and Schultz *et al.* (1957).

cytic cytoplasm (Fig. 79, left) terminate in profusion upon, and are applied directly to, a large proportion, perhaps half, of the surface membrane of a neuron soma and its dendrites. From such observations, the astrocytic glia, appear to provide a direct metabolic bridge between circulating blood plasma and neuronal cytoplasm; and give every appearance of being capable of modifying neuronal biochemistry.

Within the neuron and, more particularly, within its characteristic Nissl substance, Pallade and Palay (1955) have identified an interlacing endoplasmic reticulum, on the membrane profiles of which, ribonucleic acid (RNA) granules or ribosomes, are present in greater concentration than in any other cells of the body, except for the exocrine gland cells of the pancreas and the developing ovum (Fig. 80, left). At the right of Figure 80, Pappas and Purpura's (1961) electron photomicrographs of synaptic relations between neurons show pre-synaptic terminals upon dendrites. Within each axonal terminal, mitochondria and synaptic vesicles are conspicuous (above) while, within the post-synaptic cytoplasm (below), it can be observed that part of the thickening of the sub-synaptic membrane is contributed by RNA-bearing profiles of endothelial reticulum, reaching up to just below the surface in this sub-synaptic, receptor region of the post-synaptic neuron.

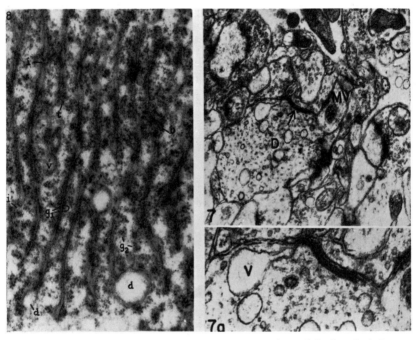

Fig. 80. Electron micrograph (*left*) of section of Nissl body of abducens motor neuron, showing profusion of RNA granules lining membranes of endoplasmic reticulum and scattered through the adjacent cytoplasm. From Palay and Palade (1955). Electron micrographs (*right, above*) of the cortical neuropile, showing a number of axo-dendritic synapses, with mito-chondria and synaptic vesicles in pre-synaptic terminals. In the enlargement (*right, below*), profiles and cisterns of endoplasmic reticulum are abundant in the cytoplasm of the post-synaptic dendrite and contribute to the density of the sub-synaptic junction. From Pappas and Purpura (1961).

RNA AND MEMORY

At a symposium of the American Psychological Association in 1947, Katz and Halstead (1950) made one of the earlier of a number of proposals that alterations in neural protein metabolism subserve the memory process; and such a view was elaborated further by McCulloch (1950) in 1949 at a Macy Conference on Cynerbetics, which he chaired. The Zeitgeist of that period was not a favorable one, however, for such enlightened views. On the one hand, the behavioral iconoclasts nihilistically held that no tangible neural region or process could account for the engram. On the other, the axon-physiologists of the '40's proposed, with simple faith, that the nerve impulse provided an adequate model for all functions of the brain. In that now-distant era, the multiplication of nerve impulses by reverberating circuits, along with plastic changes at synapses, involving swelling, outgrowth or multiplication of pre-synaptic terminals, were more attractive conceptually than prospects of modification of neural protein chemistry.

The more recent nucleic-acid studies of genetic biochemistry have, however, reopened this possibility in a most dramatic way. The Watson-Crick (1953) model of the macromolecule, de-oxyribo-nucleic acid or DNA (Fig. 81), was presented in 1953, with the conclusion "We feel that our proposed structure for DNA may help to solve one of the fundamental problems of biology—the molecular basis of the template needed for genetic replication." It now appears likely that, in addition, such a model may provide a molecular basis for the formation and preservation of memory as well (Schmitt, 1962). Subsequent work has revealed the mutable capacity of DNA molecules, in which the order or configuration of constituent links of amino-acid residues, often called the genetic code, can undergo alterations which, once induced, can be serially reconstituted in metabolism in identical replication. The DNA molecules of the nucleus have been determined, furthermore, to provide a template for the formation of RNA molecules which pass, like messengers, into the cytoplasm of the cell; in turn, to form templates guiding the production of the protein factories in the ribosome particles along the endothelial reticulum. All of these current advances in molecular biology relating DNA and genetic coding now seem potentially applicable to memory coding, in terms of analogous modification of neuronal RNA.

Cytochemical studies of neural RNA have been undertaken by Hydén (1959, 1960) in individual nerve cells, which he has

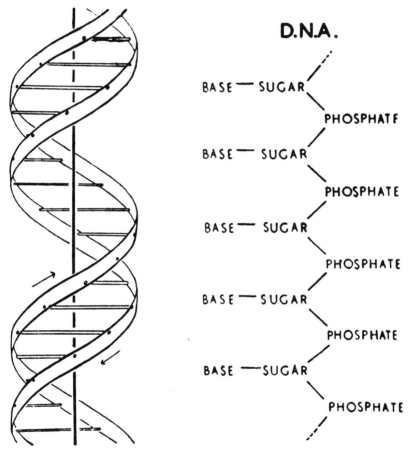

Fig. 81. The Watson-Crick model of desoxyribonucleic acid (*left*) shows a pair of DNA chains wound, as a double helix, around a central axis. At the right is the phosphate-sugar backbone of each chain, from each unit of which protrudes a base, linked to an opposing base in the opposite chain. The sequence of these bases forms the genetic code. From Watson and Crick (1953).

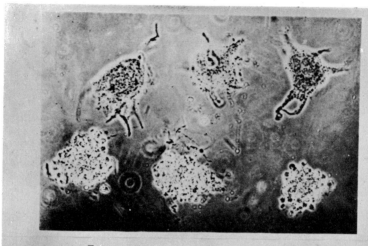

THE EFFECT OF STIMULATION ON THE RNA OF DEITERS' NERVE CELLS
AND GLIAL CELLS
RNA content ($\mu\mu$g/cell) from controls and from rabbits stimulated 25 min/day for
7 days. In all 26 animals were used. Notation as in Table 1.

		N	RNA content (mean)	*V*	*P*
Deiters' nerve cell	Stimulated	105	1612	11	0·01**
	Controls	114	1545	12	
Glial cells	Stimulated	30	85	22	0·001***
	Controls	25	123	35	

N = number of cells analysed
V = the coefficient of variation, $\frac{s \times 100}{\text{mean}}$
P = probability after *t*-test

Fig. 82. Three nerve cells from Deiter's nucleus (*above*), cleared of their surrounding glia (*below*) and photographed with phase-contrast microscopy. The table (*below*) shows the RNA gain by neurons, matched by an RNA loss in glial cells, as a consequence of vestibular stimulation preceding sacrifice. From Hydén and Pigon (1960).

been able to dissect from Deiter's vestibular nucleus in the rabbit brain and strip of their surrounding glia (Fig. 82, above). Analysis of such cells in control states and following stimulation, induced by rotating the animals before sacrifice (Hydén and Pigon, 1960) reveal a high resting level of neuronal RNA, as well as its increment in the nerve cell, and concomitant depletion in glia, as a consequence of physiological stimulation (Fig. 82, below). Such findings have led Hydén to suggest that the neuron and its glia form a kind of functional micromodule, in which the glial element acts as a biochemical and energy donator for the neuron.

Hydén (1960) has extended these possibilities to the formation of an hypothesis of a memory mechanism, whose successive stages (Fig. 83, left to right) propose that there is: first, a specification of cytoplasmic RNA in the neuron, as a consequence of glial-neural excitation; second, this altered or specified RNA provides a template for the formation of specific amino-acid sequences in the subsequent production of proteins; third, dissociation of this specific protein activates transmitter substances in a pattern like that initially induced; and last, these transmitter substances excite the post-synaptic cell. More generally, the RNA which has once been specified by a characteristic pattern

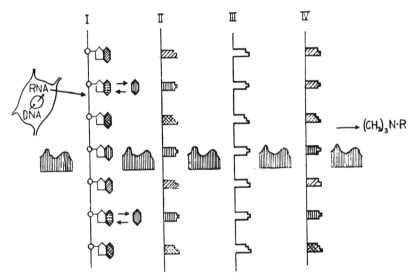

Fig. 83. Hydén's hypothesis of a memory mechanism proposes that DNA directs protein production in the cytoplasm via RNA (*left*). In successive stages, to the *right*: (1) RNA specification, through modulated frequencies of neural-glial excitation, produces (II) specified protein, which (III) becomes activated by combination with a complementary molecule, and (IV) releases transmitter substances which excite the post-synaptic cell. From Hydén (1960).

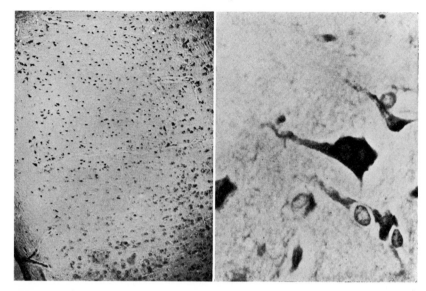

Fig. 84. Photomicrograph of section through rabbit cortex (*left*), showing
mirror focus, in which dark staining marks an increase of RNA, following
bombardment from seizurogenic lesion of opposite hemisphere. In high
magnification (*right*), the positive staining RNA is seen to be concentrated
along the inner surface of the soma membrane and extends out into the
dendrite. From Morrell (1961).

of neuronal excitation is proposed to continue to replicate itself
and to respond to this same excitatory pattern whenever it is repeated, but not to other patterns of excitation.

Hydén's (1960) hypothesis thus conceives of an intracellular
neuronal mechanism for information storage in terms of induced
molecular specificity. It is based on the principle that nucleo-
protein production is as characteristic and as functionally significant for neurons, as is impulse production and propagation.
It holds, in short, that nucleo-protein production is augmented
by increasing neuronal activity and that the protein so produced
display biochemical specificity, continue to replicate their
changed configuration, and become reactivated functionally by
the same circumstances as those initially setting them into play.

Support for this hypothesis has recently been provided by
observation of an increase in neural RNA induced by trans-
synaptic bombardment of pyramidal cells within the cerebral

cortex of the brain. Morrell (1961) established an epileptic focus in one cerebral hemisphere of the rabbit's brain, following which maintained discharge to the mirror area of the opposite hemisphere led finally to an increase of cytoplasmic RNA, displayed by specific cytochemical staining (Fig. 84). Morrell (1961) comments, "Since the cells of the mirror focus have been shown to have some of the attributes of learning and of memory, it is perhaps not too far-fetched to consider that the complex of ribonucleic acid and protein represents an essential element in the molecular basis of memory."

These studies and concepts point to new directions in which research toward applied goals might profitably move. If the nucleic acid configuration of neural cytoplasm can be changed by use, in a LaMarckian kind of fashion, and this alteration is preserved and replicated during metabolism and can continue to influence performance on a long-term basis, it might be possible to gain biochemical or pharmacological control of such alterations and manipulate them for therapeutic purposes.

Recent studies by McConnell, Jacobson and Kimble (1959), with the flatworm, Planaria, indicate that after learned behavior is acquired by training, and the animal is surgically divided, the regenerating parts continue to preserve this learning. Extension of this work by Corning and John (1961) suggests that this preservation of learning may depend upon retention and replication of specified RNA; for regenerating parts reared in a medium containing RNA-ase, an enzyme destroying RNA, do not retain earlier acquired learning, although they can subsequently be retrained. Other current work by McConnell, Jacobson and Humphries (1961) indicates that naïve, uneducated Planaria may be able to acquire learned behavior simply by cannibalizing previously trained or educated animals, presumably by oral ingestion of their specified RNA. It is intriguing to wonder whether these current experiments with flatworms are likely to form templates for future chemotherapeutic advances in medicine and, possibly, in education as well.

REFERENCES

Adey, W. R.: Brain mechanisms and the learning process. *Fed. Proc., 20:* 617-627, 1961.

Adey, W. R., Dunlop, C. W. and Sunderland, S.: A survey of rhinocephalic interconnections with the brain stem. *J. Comp. Neurol., 110:*173-203, 1958.

Adey, W. R., Dunlop, C. W. and Hendrix, C. E.: Hippocampal slow waves, distribution and phase relationships in the course of approach learning. *AMA Arch. Neurol., 3:*74-90, 1960.

Adey, W. R., Walter, D. O. and Hendrix, C. E.: Computer techniques in correlation and spectral analyses of cerebral slow waves during discriminative behavior. *Exp. Neurol., 3:*501-524, 1961.

Brazier, M. A. B.: Long-persisting electrical traces in the brain of man and their possible relationship to higher nervous activity. Pp. 347-358. In Jasper, H. H. and Smirnov, G. D. (Eds.) *The Moscow Colloquium on EEG and Higher Nervous Activity. EEG Clin. Neurophysiol.* Suppl. 13, 1960.

Brown, S. and Schäfer, E. A.: An investigation into the functions of the occipital and temporal lobes of the monkey's brain. *Phil. Trans. Roy. Soc. Lond., B, 179:*303-327, 1888.

Bureš, J. Reversible decortication and behavior. Pp. 234-242. In Brazier, M. A. B. (Ed.) *CNS and Behavior,* New York, 1959.

Corning, W. C. and John, E. R.: Effect of ribonuclease on retention of conditioned response in regenerated planarians. *Science 134:*1363-1365, 1961.

Deutsch, J. A.: Higher nervous function: the physiological bases of memory. *Ann. Rev. Physiol., 24:*259-286, 1962.

Doty, R. W., Beck, E. C. and Kovi, K. A.: Effect of brain-stem lesions on conditioned responses of cats. *Exp. Neurol., 1:*360-385, 1959.

Feindel, W. and Penfield, W.: Localization of discharge in temporal lobe automatism. *AMA Arch. Neurol. Psychiat., 72:*605-630, 1954.

Galambos, R.: A glia-neural theory of brain function. *Proc. Nat. Acad. Sci., 47:*129-136, 1961.

Gerard, R. W.: Biological roots of psychiatry. *Science, 122:*225-230, 1955.

Green, J. D.: Some recent electrophysiological and electron microscope studies of Ammon's horn. Pp. 266-271. In Tower, D. B. and Schadé, J. P. (Eds.) *Structure and Function of the Cerebral Cortex,* Elsevier, Amsterdam, 1959.

Green, J. D. and Adey, W. R.: Electrophysiological studies of hippocampal connections and excitability. *EEG Clin. Neurophysiol., 8:*245-262, 1956.

Green, J. D. and Arduini, A.: Hippocampal electrical activity in arousal. *J. Neurophysiol., 17:*533-557, 1954.

Green, J. D., Maxwell, D. S., Schindler, W. J. and Stumpf, C.: Rabbit EEG "theta" rhythm: its anatomical source and relation to activity in single neurons. *J. Neurophysiol., 23:*403-420, 1960.

Hernandez-Péon, R. and Brust-Carmona, H.: Functional role of subcortical structures in habituation and conditioning. Pp. 393-408. In Delafresnaye, J. F. (Ed.) *Brain Mechanisms and Learning,* Blackwell, Oxford, 1961.

Hild, W. and Tasaki, I.: Morphological and physiological properties of neurons and glial cells in tissue culture. *J. Neurophysiol.*, 25:277-304, 1962.

Hughlings Jackson, J.: On a particular variety of epilepsy (intellectual aura), one case with symptoms of organic brain disease. *Brain*, 11: 179-207, 1888.

Hydén, H.: Biochemical changes in glial cells and nerve cells at varying activity. In Brücke, F. (Ed.): *Biochemistry of the Central Nervous System.* Symp. III. Proc. 4th. Internat. Mtg. Biochem. vol. 3, pp. 64-89, Pergamon Press, London, 1959.

Hydén, H.: The neuron. Chap. 5. Pp. 215-323. In: Bracket, J. and Mirsky, A. E. (Eds.) *The Cell.* Vol. 5. Academic Press, N.Y., 1960.

Hydén, H. and Pigon, A.: A cytophysiological study of the functional relationship between oligo-dendroglial cells and nerve cells of Deiter's nucleus. *J. Neurochem.*, 6:57-72, 1960.

Ingram, W. R.: Modification of learning by lesions and stimulation in the diencephalon and related structures. Pp. 535-544. In Jasper, H. H. (Ed.) *Reticular Formation of the Brain*, Little Brown, Boston, 1958.

Jowett, B.: *The Dialogues of Plato.* Vol. IV. *Theaetetus*, p. 254. Oxford Univ. Press, 1931.

Jung, R. and Kornmüller, A. E.: Eine Methodik der Ableitung lokalisierten Potentialschwankungen aus subcorticalen Hirngebeiten. *Arch. f. Psych. u. Nervenkr.*, 109:1-30, 1938.

Kaada, B. R., Rasmussen, E. W. and Kveim, O.: Effects of hippocampal lesions on maze learning and retention in rats. *Exp. Neurol.*, 3:333-355, 1961.

Katz, J. J. and Halstead, W. C.: Protein organization and mental function pp. 1-38. In Halstead, W. C. (Ed.) *Brain and Behavior. A Symposium. Comp. Physiol. Monographs* v. 20, No. 1. Univ. Calif. Press, 1950.

King, F. A.: Effects of septal and amygdaloid lesions on emotional behavior and conditioned avoidance responses in the rat. *J. Nerv. Ment. Dis.*, 126:57-63, 1958.

Klüver, H. and Bucy, P. L.: Preliminary analysis of functions of the temporal lobes in monkeys. *Arch. Neurol. Psychiat.*, 42:979-1000, 1939.

Korsakow, S. S.: Über eine besondere Form psychische Störung, combinirt mit multipler Neuritis. *Arch. f. Phychiat.*, 21:669-704, 1890.

Liberson, W. T. and Cadhilac, J. G.: Electroshock and rhinencephalic seizure states. *Confinia Neurol.*, 13:278-286, 1953.

Mahut, H.: Effects of subcortical electrical stimulation on learning in the rat. *Am. Psychol.*, 12:466, 1957.

Maynard, E. A., Schultz, R. L. and Pease, D. C.: Electron microscopy of the vascular bed of rat cerebral cortex. *Am. J. Anat.*, 100:409-434, 1957.

McConnell, J. V., Jacobson, A. L. and Kimble, D. P.: The effects of regeneration upon retention of a conditioned response in the planarian. *J. Comp. Physiol. Psychol.*, 52:1-5, 1959.

McCulloch, W.: Introductory discussion, pp. 13-17. In Foerster, H. von (Ed.) *Cybernetics*. Josiah Macy, Jr. Found., New York, 1950.

Milner, B.: Psychological defects produced by temporal lobe incision. Chap. VII. In *The Brain and Human Behavior. Res. Pub. Assn. Nerv. Ment. Dis.*, 36:244-257, 1958.

Mitarai, G., Svaetichin, G., Vallecalle, E., Fatehchand, R., Villegas, J. and Laufer, M.: Glia-neuron interactions and adaptional mechanism of the retina. Pp. 463-481. In: Jung, R. (Ed.) *The Visual System: Neurophysiology and Psychophysics*. Springer-Verlag, Berlin, 1961.

Morrell, F.: Lasting changes in synaptic organization produced by continuous neuronal bombardment. Pp. 375-392. In Dalafresnaye, J. F.: (Ed.) *Brain Mechanisms and Learning*, Blackwell, Oxford, 1961.

Olds, J. and Olds, M. E.: Interference and learning in paleocortical systems. Pp. 153-187. In Delafresnaye, J. F. (Ed.) *Brain Mechanisms and Learning*, Blackwell, Oxford, 1961.

Orbach, J., Milner, B. and Rasmussen, T.: Learning and retention in monkeys after amygdala-hippocampus resection. *Arch. Neurol.*, 3:230-251, 1960.

Palay, S. L. and Palade, G. E.: The fine structure of neurons. *J. Biophys. Biochem. Cytol.*, 1:69-88, 1955.

Pappas, G. D. and Purpura, D. P.: Fine structure of dendrites in the superficial neocortical neuropile. *Exper. Neurol.*, 4:507-530, 1961.

Penfield, W.: The interpretive cortex. *Science, 129*:1719-1725, 1959.

Penfield, W. and Milner, B.: Memory deficit produced by bilateral lesions in the hippocampal zone. *AMA Arch. Neurol. Psychiat., 79*:475-497, 1958.

Petsche, H., Stumpf, C. and Gogolak, G.: The significance of the rabbit's septum as a relay station between the midbrain and hippocampus. *EEG Clin. Neurophysiol., 14*:202-211, 1962.

Schmitt, F. O. (Ed.): *Macromolecular Specificity and Biological Memory*. M.I.T. Press, Cambridge, 1962.

Schultz, R. L., Maynard, E. A. and Pease, D. C.: Electron microscopy of neurons and neuroglia of cerebral cortex and corpus collosum. *Am. J. Anat., 100*:369-408, 1957.

Scoville, W. B.: The limbic lobe in man. *J. Neurosurg., 11*:64-66, 1954.

Stamm, J. S. and Pribram, K. H.: Effects of epileptogenic lesions of inferotemporal cortex on learning and retention in monkeys. *J. Comp. Physiol. Psychol., 54*:614-618, 1961.

Stepien, L. S., Cordeau, J. P. and Rasmussen, T.: The effect of temporal lobe and hippocampal lesions on auditory and visual recent memory in monkeys. *Brain, 83*:470-489, 1960.

Svaetichin, G., Laufer, M., Mitarai, G., Fatechand, R., Vallecalle, E. and Villegas, J.: Glial control of neuronal networks and receptors. Pp. 445-456. In Jung, R. and Kornhuber, H. *The Visual System*. Springer, Berlin, 1961.

Talland, G. A.: Psychological studies of Korsakoff's psychosis: VI Memory and learning. *J. Nerv. Ment. Dis., 130:*366-385, 1960.

Thompson, R.: The effect of intracranial stimulation on memory in cats. *J. Comp. Physiol. Psychol., 51:*421-426, 1958.

Victor, M., Angevine, J. B., Mancall, E. L. and Fisher, C. M.: Memory loss with lesions of hippocampal formation. *Arch. Neurol., 5:*244-263, 1961.

Watson, J. D. and Crick, F. H. C.: Genetical implications of the structure of deoxyribonucleic acid. *Nature, 171:*964-967, 1953.

9

BRAIN MECHANISMS FOR INTERNAL INHIBITION AND LIGHT SLEEP

Sɪɢɴɪғɪᴄᴀɴᴛ ᴀᴛᴛᴇɴᴛɪᴏɴ ᴛᴏ ɪɴʜɪʙɪᴛɪᴏɴ, in the neurophysiological sense, dates from 1845, when the Webers (Fulton, 1930) reported that vagal excitation slowed or stopped the heart. Some years later, in 1862, Sechenov (Subkov, 1935) blocked spinal reflexes by stimulating the frog's brain and so discovered central neural inhibition (Fig. 5). A generation later, a young medical graduate at St. Petersburg, Pavlov, was influenced by reading Sechenov's (1866) *Reflexes of the Brain* and began research on the neural control of visceral function. Around 1900, Pavlov became attracted by psychic influences upon salivary and gastric secretion and initiated study of higher nervous activity involved in the formation and modification of conditional reflexes. In this work, Pavlov (Anrep, 1927; Gantt, 1928, 1941) first identified internal inhibition. By appropriate experimental procedures, he found it possible both to induce conditioned responses and additionally, to establish "a learning not to respond." This cessation of performance, effected as a consequence of prior experience, was called internal inhibition, to distinguish it from external inhibition, typified by cessation of behavior when strong, novel, extraneous stimulation evokes an orienting reflex (see page 112).

In an alert and active dog responding regularly to signals in a Pavlovian camera, a striking behavioral change follows induction of internal inhibition. Secreto-motor responses gradually diminish and cease. Drowsiness and lassitude develop and become more and more profound. If the process is pushed to the extreme, the eyes close, the head droops, the body relaxes and hangs on the loops of the stand, as the animal passes into sleep and emits an occasional snore. Pavlov conceived that the biological significance of this process lay in its ability to perfect the signalizing and analyzing activities of the brain, making possible more effective adaptation to the environment. Additionally, he proposed that internal inhibition provided opportunity for refreshment and recovery, after excitation and fatigue. Upon irradiating and becoming generalized in the brain, it was responsible, he held, for sleep. In the latter part of his long career, when Pavlov attempted to apply his laboratory findings to psychiatry, he suggested that some types of mental illness might be explicable in terms of abnormal internal inhibition.

THALAMO-CORTICAL MECHANISM FOR INTERNAL INHIBITION

Following Pavlov's contributions, two succeeding discoveries have been of greatest significance for the proposal that a diffusely projecting, thalamo-cortical, EEG-synchronizing system constitutes the neural mechanism of internal inhibition. The first of these, by Hess (1944), reported the induction of behavioral sleep by low-frequency, electrical stimulation of the paramedial thalamic region of the cat (Fig. 85). Later EEG studies, by Hess, Jr., Koella and Akert (1953) and by Akimoto and his associates (1956), showed this induced sleep to be associated with large-amplitude, slow waves and spindle bursts characteristic of light sleep, both in animals and in man.

In a second major contribution, Morison and Dempsey (1942) and Dempsey and Morison (1942, 1943) found that low-frequency stimulation of this midline thalamic region evoked a progressively recruiting, wave-like response in the cortical EEG (Figs. 51, 86, 99). These widely distributed recruiting responses resembled spontaneous spindle bursts, and the two interacted with one another; contrastingly, no interaction occurred with focal cortical discharge, evoked by peripheral afferent stimulation. From their studies, Morison and Dempsey proposed the existence of a nonspecific thalamo-cortical system, arising from mid-line and intralaminar nuclei, distinct from specific afferent projections of the relay thalamic nuclei (Fig. 87, left). Subsequently, Jasper and Droogleever-Fortuyn (1947) were able to evoke spike-wave discharge from this thalamo-cortical system

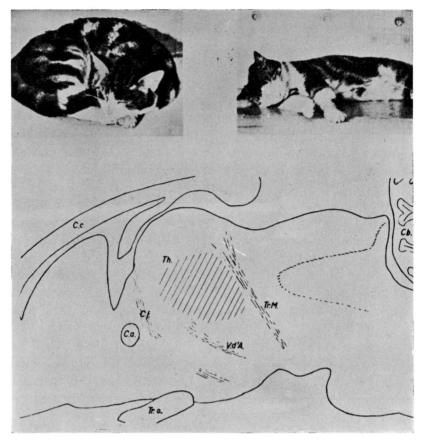

Fig. 85. Behavioral sleep induced by low frequency thalamic stimulation (*above*), with the effective medial thalamic zone marked (*below*) by shading on a parasagittal section of the cat's brain stem. From Hess (1944).

and suggested its relation to seizures of the *petit mal* type, in which loss of consciousness forms the primary symptom.

Most recently, Tissot and Monnier (1959) and Monnier and his associates (1960) have identified dual and reciprocally antagonistic components within the nonspecific thalamo-cortical projection itself (Fig. 87, right). One of these, capable of firing at rapid stimulus frequencies, forms a relay for ascending reticular influences leading to EEG arousal (see page 79); while the second, which fires best at low stimulus frequencies, is responsible for recruiting responses, spindle bursts, and synchronization of the EEG.

BULBAR DRIVING OF THALAMO-CORTICAL SYSTEM

It has recently been found possible to drive this latter, EEG-synchronizing, thalamo-cortical mechanism experimentally from a number of other regions of the brain. A profusion of recent studies has shown that this system can be driven from the bulbo-pontile levels of the brainstem. Baroreceptor stimulation, leading to syncope and other inhibitory effects, has been shown by Bonvallet, Dell and Hiebel (1954) and Dell and his associates (1961) to be associated with generalized synchronization of the EEG. In agreement, Moruzzi and his associates (1960) have evoked large slow waves and spindle bursts in the EEG by low-frequency stimulation of the solitary tract and bulbo-reticular formation. When this bulbar synchronizing mechanism is eliminated by transection through the pons or by reversible pharmaco-

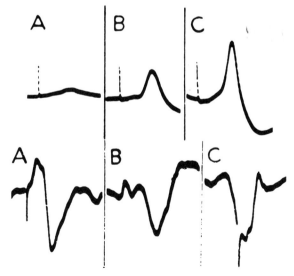

Fig. 86. Cortical recruiting responses (*above*) evoked by 8/sec. stimulation of the nonspecific thalamo-cortical system. Recruiting response (A, *below*) and wave of spontaneous spindle burst (B) resemble one another and interact (C), recruiting response cannot be elicited immediately after a burst wave. From Morison and Dempsey (1942).

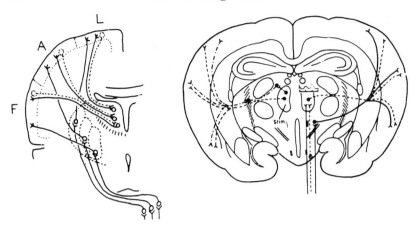

Fig. 87. Diagram (*left*) showing independence of specific afferent and nonspecific thalamo-cortical projections. From Morison and Dempsey (1942). Diagram (*right*) showing further independence of nonspecific thalamo-cortical system for recruiting responses and EEG synchronization (*left*), from that relaying ascending reticular influences for EEG arousal (*right*). From Tissot and Monnier (1959).

logical block (Moruzzi, 1960), an initially synchronized EEG gives way to a pattern of EEG arousal (Fig. 88). This bulbo-pontile, EEG synchronizing and internally-inhibiting influence, capable of interoceptor excitation, would seem from its lowly position to be phylogenetically old. Possibly it is directed toward influencing visceral function generally through the body by reducing the excitability of the brain.

SATIETY AND INTERNAL INHIBITION

Other mechanisms capable of driving the synchronizing thalamo-cortical system are present in the hypothalamus, where they appear to be related to the regulation of innate behavior and to the control of pituitary secretion. In a study of the neuro-endocrine control of sexual behavior, Sawyer and Kawakami (1959) and Kawakami and Sawyer (1959) have observed a period of several minutes following coitus, in which the female rabbit displays a languid relaxation and inactivity, resembling internal inhibition, which terminates abruptly in a rebound burst of feeding (Fig. 89). During this period, the animal's EEG first

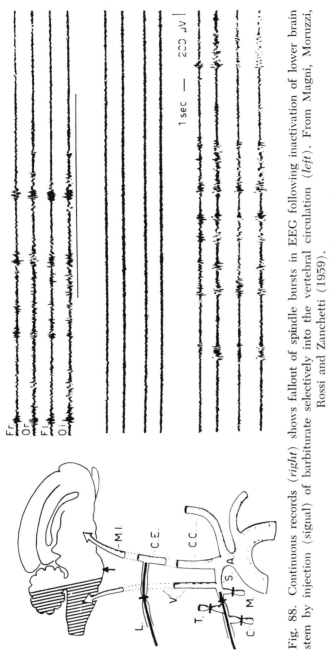

Fig. 88. Continuous records (*right*) shows fallout of spindle bursts in EEG following inactivation of lower brain stem by injection (signal) of barbiturate selectively into the vertebral circulation (*left*). From Magni, Moruzzi, Rossi and Zanchetti (1959).

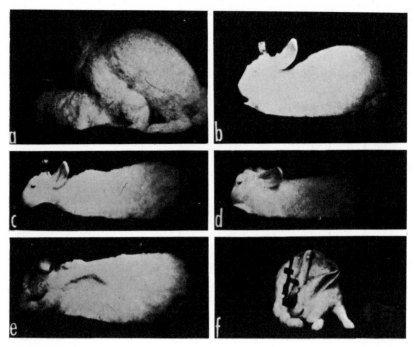

Fig. 89. Serial photos showing reduction of behavior in the female rabbit following coitus (a). In (b), the eyes close and at this time frontal spindle bursts appear. In (c-e), the head sinks to the floor, the ears droop and behavioral depression is complete; at this time, the EEG is that of paradoxical sleep, and hippocampal hypersynchrony is pronounced. In (f), the animal suddenly recovers and feeds ravenously for a few moments.
From Sawyer and Kawakami (1961).

displays cortical spindle bursts, followed by the pattern of paradoxical sleep (see page 179), associated with a prodigious hypersynchrony in limbic structures. In a primed rabbit, the administration of gonadotrophic hormones leads to a similar inhibition of behavior, which is likewise accompanied by the EEG changes just described.

There is indication that adrenocortical, as well as gonadal hormones may influence the thalamo-cortical, EEG synchronizing mechanism, for Feldman, Todt and Porter (1961) have shown that responses evoked in this midline thalamic system by afferent stimulation become increased progressively after intravenous injection of hydrocortisone (Fig. 90). Such endocrine potentiation of this mechanism suggests that an elevated titer of target gland hormones in the circulation of the brain may, by promoting internal inhibition, reduce the activity of hypothalamic neural systems initiating the secretion of pituitary trophic hormones. If so, this mechanism may form the basis for the negative feedback control of pituitary function (Fig. 22), in which there is increasingly compelling evidence for the presence of a central neural stage.

In the study of feeding behavior, Anokhin (1961) has observed an EEG arousal pattern in the frontal cortex and hypothalamus of dogs, hungry from deprivation of food. When food is tubed directly into the stomach of these hungry animals, and glucose injected into their bloodstream, this EEG arousal pattern gives way promptly to a record of pronounced synchrony both in cortical and hypothalamic channels (Fig. 91). Both feeding and sexual activity are initiated by appetites and terminated by what has been called satiety. In showing how their termination—in inactivity, lassitude, drowsiness and often sleep—is associated with synchrony and spindle bursting in the electrical activity of the brain, these findings suggest that satiety may be the expression of a type of internal inhibition which, after consummation is achieved, plays an important role in bringing innate behavior to an end.

In its role in innate behavior, as well as in regulation of en-

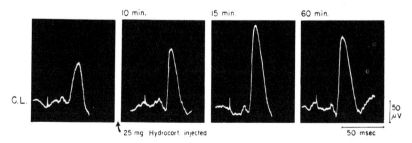

Fig. 90. Serial oscillograms show enhancement of excitability of intralaminar thalamic nucleus of cat induced by hydrocortisone. Increase in amplitude of thalamic potentials evoked by sciatic shocks appears within ten minutes after IV injection and continues for an hour. From Feldman, Todt and Porter (1961).

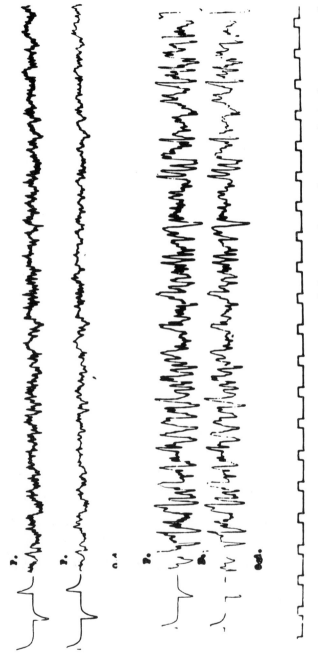

Fig. 91. Records of electrical activity of the frontal cortex of the cat under urethane anesthesia show an aroused EEG during hunger (*above*) and contrasting EEG synchrony (*below*) after glucose and filling of the stomach with milk. From Anokhin (1961).

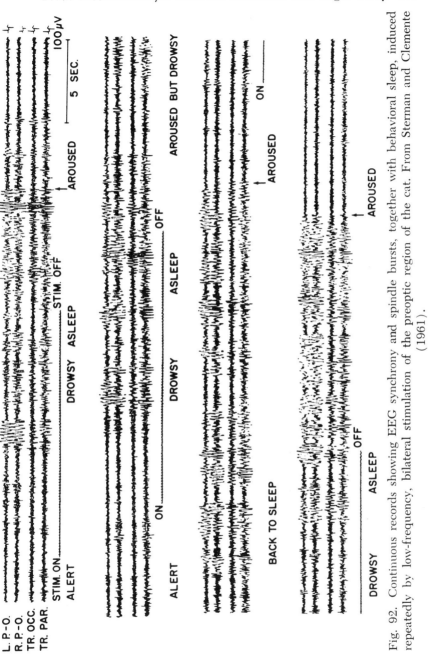

Fig. 92. Continuous records showing EEG synchrony and spindle bursts, together with behavioral sleep, induced repeatedly by low-frequency, bilateral stimulation of the preoptic region of the cat. From Sterman and Clemente (1961).

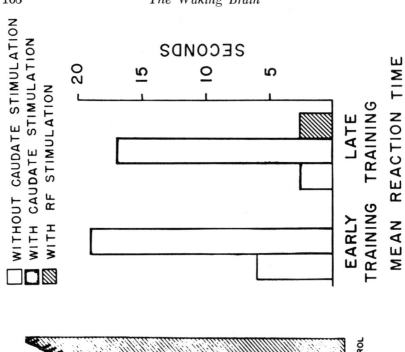

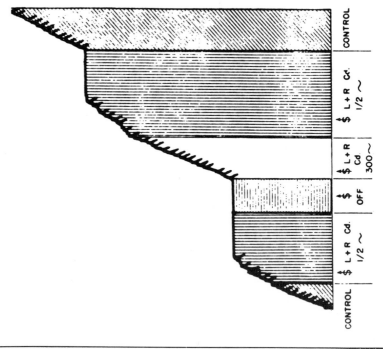

docrine and visceral function, the hypothalamus is intimately related to limbic structures of the forebrain, and is functionally connected with them through the septal and preoptic regions. (See page 62.) Recently, Sterman and Clemente (1962) have found that bilateral, low-frequency stimulation of the preoptic region is an exceedingly potent and expeditious way of inducing widespread EEG spindling and behavioral sleep (Fig. 92), and these alterations appear to be mediated by the diffuse thalamo-cortical system.

CAUDATE DRIVING OF THALAMO-CORTICAL SYSTEM

Striking effects have been obtained also from stimulating the caudate nucleus, interposed, like certain of the limbic structures, between the cerebral cortex and the stem of the brain. Buchwald and his associates (1961), extending earlier work of Akert and Andersson (1951) and of Umbach (1959), have demonstrated a caudate loop, the low-frequency-excitation of which is capable of driving the nonspecific thalamo-cortical system responsible for widespread synchronization of the EEG, with related behavioral consequences of internal inhibition, drowsiness and sleep. The influence of such caudate stimulation has been tested upon operant behavior, in which a cat pushes a lever for a food reward. As seen in Figure 93 (left), when low-frequency caudate shocks trigger spindle bursts in the EEG, lever-pushing slows and stops. Observations were also made when an animal had to discriminate between one and ten light flashes per second to obtain a food reward. Stimulation caused some impairment of accuracy but the chief consequence was a great prolongation of reaction time

←——————————————————————————————————

Fig. 93. Cumulative counter records of a cat pressing a lever for food reward (*left*). Cessation of behavior is twice induced by low-frequency, bilateral caudate shocks, which trigger spindle bursts in the EEG. High-frequency caudate stimulation restores lever-pressing. From Buchwald, Wyers, Lauprecht and Heuser (1961). Bar graphs (*right*) show marked increase of reaction time of cat's response to visual stimulation, during low-frequency stimulation of the caudate nucleus. From Buchwald, Wyers, Carlin and Farley (1961).

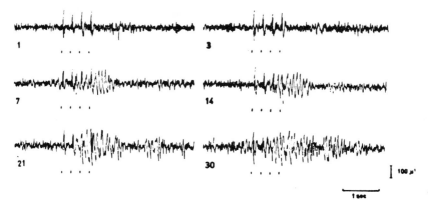

Fig. 94. Electrical activity of the visual cortex of a cat, previously conditioned to four flashes of light at 1/sec., associated with a shock to the
leg. The numbers indicate the trials without reinforcement. During extinction, note that photic stimulation increasingly triggers spindle bursts. From
Hernandez-Péon (1960).

(Fig. 93, right). During study of conditional alpha blockade (see
page 117) and visuomotor reaction time in man, Morrell and
Ross (1953) earlier observed a marked prolongation of reaction
time during the induction of Pavlovian internal inhibition by
delay, differentiation, or extinction.

INTERNAL INHIBITION OF HIGHER NERVOUS ACTIVITY

Moving sequentially up the brain, we come last to features
of higher nervous activity, in the study of which Pavlov first distinguished internal inhibition. Because of technical limitations
of that time, his studies were necessarily confined to observations
of peripheral behavior, though his conceptual insight into their
central neural mechanisms was remarkably astute. More recently,
both in Soviet and in Western neurophysiology, classical Pavlovian experiments are being repeated with concomitant recording of electrical activity of the brain (see page 116). In each of
the several categories of conditional reflex performance in which
Pavlov found internal inhibition to occur—in the inhibition of
delay, in conditioned inhibition, in differentiation and in extinc-

tion—recent electrophysiological studies have revealed features of hypersynchronization and/or spindle bursting in the EEG.

Extinction has been studied by Roitbak (1958) by observing the responses of the auditory cortex of the cat to clicks which, following training, had come to form the conditional signal for salivary secretion. During extinction, when in Pavlov's view, internal inhibition was induced, cortical click responses gained progressively in amplitude and recurring spindle bursts appeared in the EEG. In the experiments of Hernandez-Péon (1960), visual cortical responses to four flashes of light at 1/sec. were associated with a shock to the leg on the fourth flash. After a variable number of flash-shock associations, some facilitation of photic responses occurred. During subsequent extinction, bursts of slow waves were triggered by the non-reinforced photic stimuli (Fig. 94).

The work of Gluck and Rowland (1959) has explored EEG changes in the internal inhibition of delay, in which the conditional signal is prolonged for an increasingly long interval before the unconditioned stimulus is presented. During the first half of this prolongation, when Pavlov observed a cessation of the salivary secretory response, Gluck and Rowland recorded a period of synchronization and spindle bursting in the EEG. Additionally, they have performed ingenious experiments on conditioned inhibition in sleeping animals, for whom the presentation of clicks formed a conditional signal (established in earlier training during wakefulness) for a terminal electric shock to the skin. As seen in Figure 95, although the animal remains behaviorally asleep as the conditional clicks begin and continue, the sleeping EEG displays arousal changes. A tone is then presented which (again from earlier training during wakefulness) signals withholding of painful reinforcement. Shortly after this tone begins, the EEG record returns once more to the sleeping type, to arouse again upon conclusion of the tone. Last, as the warning clicks finally end, without a shock, the EEG returns to sleep and gets terminally into line with behavior.

In the work of Kogan (1960), an approach to food was conditioned to a metronome signal of 60/min, while differentiation or absence of response was developed by lack of reinforcement

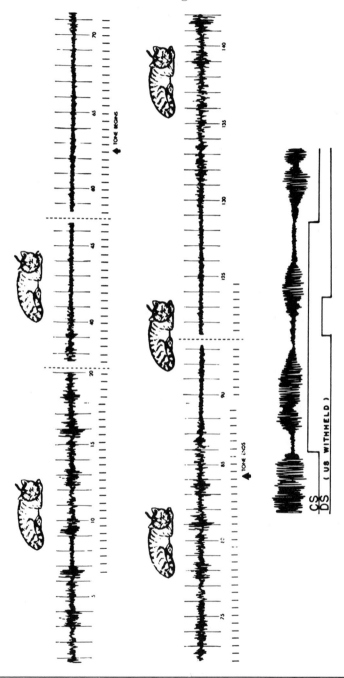

to a signal at 120/min. The latter then began to evoke extraordinary hypersynchronization instead of the customary desynchronization of the EEG from the motor cortex. In Kogan's experience, other types of internal inhibition are similarly accompanied by hypersynchronization, in which "the neurons of the vast areas of the analyzers which have been switched out of operation, are drawn together in a resting rhythm." In their EEG studies related to the differentiation of conditional signals, John and his associates (1961) have observed that while inhibition of conditional responses was consistently accompanied by slow waves, these might also occur during excitation. Records from component nuclei of the nonspecific thalamic system did not display any conspicuous features related to these changes, nor could differential inhibition be induced by frequency specific excitation of these thalamic areas. John and his associates (1961) conclude "Our data do not provide support for the suggestion that the inhibitory cortical slow waves arise as a consequence of slow activity propagated from these structures to the cortex, or vice versa."

In summation, these many contributions point to the existence of a nonspecific, thalamo-cortical system, the low-frequency excitation of which, evokes large slow waves as well as recruiting responses and spindle bursts in the EEG. These characteristically bear a close relation to internal inhibition, behavioral drowsiness and sleep, although they can display dissociation from such behavior. Differentiable components exist in this thalamo-cortical system and are capable of being driven more or less independently by inputs from a number of other parts of the brain. In-

---

Fig. 95. Continuous record of cortical electrical activity in a sleeping cat, with changes diagrammed below. Note that EEG arousal induced by presentation of the conditional stimulus (clicks, marked by vertical lines below record) is twice interrupted by spindle bursts. The first group of bursts (*upper left*) is associated with inhibition of delay, and the second (*lower left*) with presentation of a differential stimulus (tone, the onset and conclusion of which is indicated by arrows), signalling withholding of painful reinforcement. When the conditional signal ends, the EEG returns to a sleeping pattern. From Gluck and Rowland (1959).

volvement of this mechanism from bulbo-pontile sources may be designed to effect a general reduction of visceral processes. Its excitation from hypothalamic and limbic structures appears to serve a feedback control of pituitary secretion and provide a means of terminating innate behavior by satiety. When activated from the basal ganglia and cerebral cortex, this system appears to manage all the Pavlovian categories of internal inhibition of higher nervous activity, including that of sleep itself.

If the inferences drawn from these many contributions are correct, it is now possible to identify a thalamo-cortical mechanism for internal inhibition, capable of modifying activity of the brain partially or globally, so that its sensory, motor and higher functions become reduced and cease. The consequences of the action of this mechanism are the opposite of those of the ascending reticular activating system (see page 90) for internal excitation. The principle of reciprocal innervation proposed by Sherrington to account for spinal-reflex integration would appear relevant to the manner in which these two higher antagonistic neural mechanisms determine the alternating patterns of brain activity manifest as wakefulness and light sleep.

REFERENCES

Akert, K. and Andersson, B.: Experimenteller Beitrag zur Physiologie des Nucleus Caudatus. *Acta Physiol. Scand.*, 22:22-281-298, 1951.

Akimoto, H., Yamaguchi, N., Okabe, K., Nakagawa, T., Nakamura, I., Abe, K., Horli, T., and Masahashi, K.: On the sleep induced through electrical stimulation of dog thalamus. *Folia Psych. Neurol. Jap.*, 10:117-146, 1956.

Anokhin, P. K.: The multiple ascending infiuences of the subcortical centers on the cerebral cortex. In Brazier, M. A. B. (Ed.) *Brain and Behavior.* American Institute of Biological Sciences, Washington, 1961.

Batini, C., Moruzzi, G., Palestrini, M., Rossi, G. F., and Zanchetti, A.: Effects of complete pontine transections on the sleep-wakefulness rhythm: the midpontine pretrigeminal preparation. *Arch. Ital. Biol.*, 97:1-12, 1959,

Batini, C., Magni, F., Palestrini, M., Rossi, G. F. and Zanchetti, A.: Neural mechanisms underlying the enduring EEG and behavioral activation in the midpontine pretrigeminal cat. *Arch. Ital. Biol.*, 97:13-25, 1959.

Bonvallet, M., Dell, P. and Hiebel, G.: Tonus sympathique et activite electrique corticale. *EEG Clin. Neurophysiol.*, 6:119-144, 1954.

Buchwald, N. A., Wyers, E. J., Okuma, T. and Heuser, G.: The caudate spindle. 1. Electrophysiological properties. *EEG Clin. Neurophysiol., 13*:509-518, 1961.

Buchwald, N. A., Heuser, G., Wyers, E. J. and Lauprecht, C. W.: The caudate-spindle. III. Inhibition of the caudate-spindle by high frequency stimulation of subcortical structures. *EEG Clin. Neurophysiol., 13*:525-530, 1961.

Buchwald, N. A., Wyers, E. J., Lauprecht, C. W. and Heuser, G.: The caudate-spindle. IV. A behavioral index of caudate-induced inhibition. *EEG Clin. Neurophysiol., 13*:531-537, 1961.

Buchwald, N. A., Wyers, E. J., Carlin, J. and Farley, R. E.: Effects of caudate stimulation on visual discrimination. *Exp. Neurol., 4*:23-36, 1961.

Cordeau, J. P. and Mancia, M.: Evidence for the existence of an EEG synchronization mechanism originating in the lower brain stem. *EEG Clin. Neurophysiol., 11*:551-564, 1959.

Dell, P., Bonvallet, M. and Hugelin, A.: Mechanisms of reticular deactivation, pp. 86-107. In Wolstenholme, G. E. W. and O'Connor, M. (Eds.) *The Nature of Sleep.* Churchill, Ltd., London, 1961.

Dempsey, E. N. and Morison, R. S.: Interaction of certain spontaneous and induced cortical potentials. *Am. J. Physiol., 135*:301-308, 1942.

Dempsey, E. N. and Morison, R. S.: The electrical activity of a thalamo-cortical relay system. *Am. J. Physiol., 138*:283-296, 1943.

Favale, E., Loeb, C., Rossi, G. F. and Sacco, G.: EEG synchronization and Behavioral signs of sleep following low-frequency stimulation of the brain stem reticular formation. *Arch. Ital. Biol., 99*:1-22, 1961.

Feldman, S., Todt, J. C. and Porter, R. W.: Effect of adrenocortical hormones on evoked potentials in the brain stem. *Neurology, 11*:109-115, 1961.

Gluck, H. and Rowland, V.: Defensive conditioning of electrographic arousal with delayed and differentiated auditory stimuli. *EEG Clin. Neurophysiol., 11*:485-496, 1959.

Hernandez-Péon, R.: Neurophysiological correlates of habituation and other manifestations of plastic inhibition (internal inhibition). In Jasper, H. H. and Smirnov, G. D. (Eds.). *Moscow Colloquium on EEG of Higher Nervous Activity. EEG Clin. Neurophysiol. Suppl. 13,* pp. 101-114, 1960.

Hess, W. R.: Das Schlafsyndrom als Folge dienzephaler Reizung. *Helv. Physiol. Acta, 2*:305-344, 1944.

Hess, R., Jr., Koella, W. P. and Akert, K.: Cortical and subcortical recordings in natural and artificially induced sleep in cats. *EEG Clin. Neurophysiol., 5*:75-90, 1953.

Heuser, G., Buchwald, N. A. and Wyers, E. J.: The caudate-spindle. II. Facilitatory and inhibitory caudate-cortical pathways. *EEG Clin. Neurophysiol., 13*:519-524, 1961.

Jasper, H. H. and Droogleever-Fortuyn, J.: Experimental studies of the functional anatomy of petit mal epilepsy. *Res. Publ. Assoc. Nerv. Ment. Dis.*, 26:272-298, 1947.

John, E. R.: High nervous functions: brain functions and learning. *Ann. Rev. Physiol.*, 23:451-484, 1961.

John, E. R., Leiman, A. L. and Sachs, E.: An exploration of the functional relationship between EEG and differential inhibition. In Kline, N.S. (Ed.) *Pavlovian Conference on Higher Nervous Activity. Ann. N.Y. Acad. Sci.*, 92:1160-1182, 1961.

Kawakami, M. and Sawyer, C. H.: Induction of behavioral and EEG changes in the rabbit by hormone administration or brain stimulation. *Endocrin.*, 65:631-643, 1959.

Kawakami, M. and Sawyer, C. H.: Neuroendocrine correlates of changes in brain activity thresholds by sex steroids and pituitary hormones. *Endocrin.*, 65:652-668, 1959.

Kogan, A. B.: The manifestations of processes of higher nervous activity in the electrical potentials of the cortex during free behavior of animals. In Jasper, H. H. and Smirnov, G. D. (Eds.) *Moscow Colloquium on EEG of Higher Nervous Activity. EEG Clin. Neurophysiol.*, Suppl. 13, pp. 51-64, 1960.

Magnes, J., Moruzzi, G. and Pompeiano, D.: Electroencephalogram-synchronizing structures in the lower brain stem. In Wolstenholme, G. E. W. and O'Connor, M. (Eds.) *The Nature of Sleep*, Churchill Ltd., London, pp. 57-85, 1961.

Magni, F., Moruzzi, G., Rossi, G. F. and Zanchetti, A.: EEG arousal following inactivation of lower brain stem by selective injection of barbiturate into the vertebral circulation. *Arch. ital. Biol.*, 97:33-46, 1959.

Monnier, M., Kalbere, M. and Krupp, P.: Functional antagonism between diffuse reticular and intralaminary recruiting projections in the medial thalamus. *Exp. Neurol.*, 2:271-289, 1960.

Morison, R. S. and Dempsey, E. W.: A study of thalamo-cortical relations. *Am. J. Physiol.*, 135:281-292, 1942.

Morrell, F. and Ross, M. H.: Central inhibition in cortical conditioned reflexes. *AMA Arch. Neurol. & Psychiat.*, 70:611-616, 1953.

Moruzzi, G.: Synchronizing influences of the brain stem and the inhibitory mechanisms underlying the production of sleep by sensory stimulation. In Jasper, H. H. and Smirnov, G. D. (Eds.) *Moscow Colloquium on EEG and Higher Nervous Activity. EEG Clin. Neurophysiol. Suppl.* 13, pp. 231-257, 1960.

Pavlov, I. P.: *Conditioned Reflexes. An Investigation of the Physiological Activity of the Cerebral Cortex*. Trans. and edited by Anrep, G. V., Oxford University Press, London, 1928.

Pavlov, I. P.: *Lectures on Conditioned Reflexes*. Trans. and edited by Gantt, W. H., 2 volumes. Internat. Publ., New York, 1928, 1941.

Roitbak, A. I.: Concerning the mechanism of extinction of orientation and conditioned reflexes. *Physiol. Bohemoslovenica*, 7:125-134, 1958.

Roitbak, A. I.: Electrical phenomena in the cerebral cortex during the extinction of orientation and conditioned reflexes. In Jasper, H. H. and Smirnov, G. D. (Eds.) *Moscow Colloquium on EEG of Higher Nervous Activity. EEG Clin. Neurophysiol. Suppl. 13*, pp. 91-100, 1960.

Sawyer, C. H. and Kawakami, M.: Characteristics of behavioral and electroencephalographic after-reactions to copulation and vaginal stimulation in the female rabbit. *Endocrinol.*, 65:622-630, 1959.

Sechenov, I. M.: *Physiologische Studien über die Hemmungsmechanismen für Reflexthätigkeit des Ruckenmarks im Gehirne des Frosches*. Hirschwald, Berlin, 1863.

Sechenov, I. M.: *Reflexes of the Brain* (1866). In *Selected Works*, trans. by Subkov, A. A., State Pub. House for Biol. & Med. Lit., Moscow, 1935.

Sterman, M. B. and Clemente, C. D.: Forebrain inhibiting mechanisms; cortical synchronization induced by basal forebrain stimulation. *Exp. Neurol.*, 6:91-102, 1962; *ibid.*: Sleep patterns induced by basal forebrain stimulation in the behaving cat. *Exp. Neurol.*, 6:103-117, 1962.

Tissot, R. and Monnier, M.: Dualité du systeme thalamique de projection diffuse. *EEG Clin. Neurophysiol.*, 11:675-686, 1959.

Umbach, W.: Zur Elektrophysiologie des Caudatum der Katze. *Arch. f. Psychiat. u. Zeit. f. d. ges. Neurol.*, 199:553-572, 1959.

Weber, E. H. and E.: Experiments which prove that the vagus nerves, stimulated with a rotary electromagnetic apparatus, slow and interrupt the heart beat (1845). In Fulton, J. F., *Selected Readings in the History of Physiology*. Thomas, Springfield, Illinois, 1930.

10

DEEP SLEEP

In broad view, our daily existence can be divided into recurring periods of fundamentally opposite behavior, one of which, wakefulness, bears a cosmic relation to the lighted portion of the earth's ceaseless rotation with respect to the glowing sun. We spend the more productive and interesting two-thirds of our lives, a total of some forty to forty-five years, in a state of wakefulness. By contrast, sleep is related to the darkened portion of the earth's daily spin, in which we spend the more unproductive third of our lives, an overall total of some twenty to twenty-five years. It has been proposed that sleep may be necessary for recovery from the excitation and fatigue of wakefulness, a concept suggested more elegantly by Shakespeare (Macbeth, Act II, Sc. 2, l. 35), when he made reference to "Sleep, which knitteth up the ravelled sleeve of care."

The sleeping state is characterized by a general predominance of inactivity, within which there can be noted the breakdown of all effective relations of the individual with the external world: on the afferent side by the absence of perception and, on the efferent, by loss of capacity for most motor performance, except that maintaining vital processes. Subjective experience is not totally lacking however, for about twenty per cent of sleep is spent in dreaming, in which sequences of sensory, motor and associational activity, often strongly flavored with emotion, occur, along with rapid movements of the eyeballs and twitches of the extremities. Consolidation of such dream experiences into memory and their subsequent recall is much reduced, by comparison with subjective experience in wakefulness.

DIFFERENTIATION OF LIGHT AND DEEP SLEEP

Current study points to the existence of two differentiable stages of sleep, served by distinct neural mechanisms which appear respectively to reduce the activity of cortical and subcortical levels of the brain. The first of these is light sleep, developing from Pavlovian internal inhibition and served by the nonspecific thalamo-cortical system responsible for large amplitude slow-waves and spindle bursts characteristic of its synchronized EEG (see page 174).

A second stage of sleep, recently identified by Dement and Kleitman (1957), Dement (1958), Jouvet (1961, 1962), Rossi (1961), Hubel (1960) and others, is called deep, activated, or paradoxical sleep. It is characterized by low-voltage, fast discharge in the electrocorticogram, and by a theta rhythm in the hippocampus, which are exceedingly similar to the EEG patterns of alert wakefulness. This stage of deep sleep is never reached directly from wakefulness but only occurs after passing first through the light slow-wave thalamo-cortical stage (Figs. 96, 97). The most marked somato-vegetative changes in sleep—the complete relaxation of postural tone in the skeletal musculature,

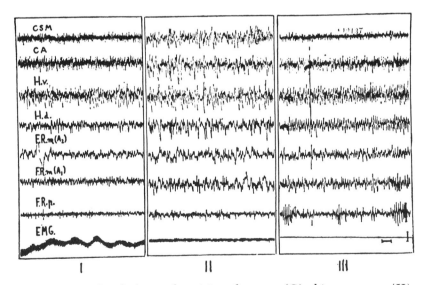

Fig. 96. Records of electrical activity of cortex (C), hippocampus (H), midbrain reticular formation (F) and electromyogram (EMG), showing patterns of activity during: I. wakefulness; II. slow wave or light sleep; III. deep or paradoxical sleep. Calibration: 1 sec. 50 μV. From Jouvet (1961).

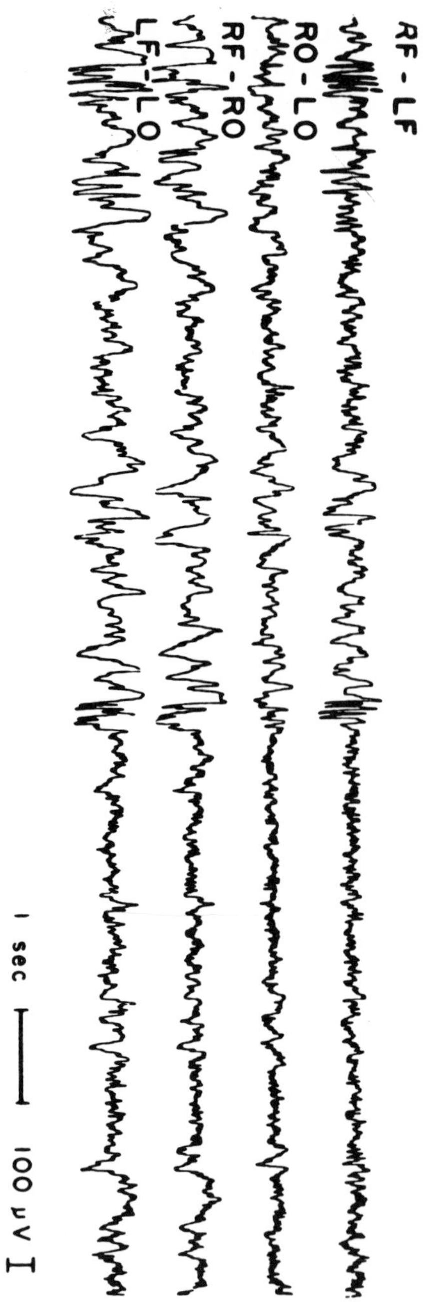
RF - LF
RO - LO
RF - RO
LF - LO
1 sec
100 µV

together with miosis, slowing of the heart and fall in blood pressure—have all been associated with this stage of deep sleep. Contrary to the earlier conclusions of Dement and Kleitman (1957), this deep, paradoxical, activated stage of sleep has recently been proposed by Jouvet (1962) to be that in which dreaming occurs.

The close resemblance of the electrocortical features of deep sleep to those of the waking EEG, is seen in Figure 97, from Hubel (1960), which also shows the characteristically rapid transition from light-slow to deep-fast sleep. The adjective "deep" applied to this stage of sleep, implies that a greater intensity of stimulation is required to induce wakefulness, whether tested by peripheral afferent stimulation or, as seen in Figure 98, from Hara *et al.* (1960), by direct, reticular stimulation, when a much higher voltage is needed to arouse an animal from the deep stage of sleep than from the light stage. Additionally, Rossi *et al.* (1961) has shown that electrocortical recruiting responses, evoked by stimulation of the nonspecific thalamic nuclei during light sleep (Fig. 99), can no longer be elicited during deep sleep. In such a situation, the induction of central barbiturate anesthesia, blocking lower brain stem function, frees the thalamocortical system, so that recruiting responses can once more be induced.

PONTILE MECHANISM FOR DEEP SLEEP

The genesis of deep sleep has been attributed by Jouvet (1961, 1962) to a source in the pontile tegmentum. Deep sleep was no longer displayed after transections of the pons and focal lesions of the medial pontile tegmentum were as effective in abolishing deep sleep as were more extensive transections (Fig. 100). When only the ponto-bulbar brain stem remained connected with the cord, the peripheral manifestations of deep sleep —the total loss of postural tone, slowing of the heart, and fall

←————————————————————————————

Fig. 97. Records of cortical electrical activity of a sleeping cat, showing rapid spontaneous transition from high voltage slow (*left*) to low voltage fast (*right*) sleep. Light sleep had begun ten minutes before; deep sleep, with twitching, continued for five minutes after the transition shown, when the animal was awakened by an auditory stimulus. From Hubel (1960).

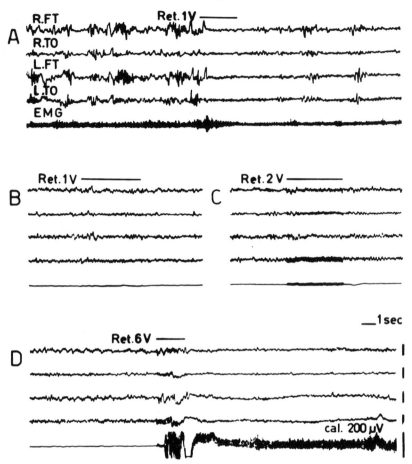

Fig. 98. Records of cortical electrical activity and EMG of a cat with stimulating electrodes implanted in the midbrain reticular formation. During light sleep (A), arousal is evoked by 1 V reticular stimulation. In B and C, 1 and 2V reticular stimulation is unable to arouse the animal from deep sleep. In D, 6V reticular stimulation awakens the animal from deep sleep, as seen best in return of tonic background in EMG. From Hara, Favale, Rossi and Sacco. (1960).

of blood pressure—continued to be manifest periodically. Jouvet proposes that ascending influences of this pontile system run forward through the ventral and medial part of the upper brain stem, independent of reticulo-cortical influences for generalized wakefulness.

GENERAL FEATURES OF LIGHT AND DEEP SLEEP

The several terms that have been used to differentiate these two stages of sleep make reference to their different distinguishing features. The terms *thalamic* and *pontile* (or rhombencephalic) sleep refer to the sites of the inhibitory mechanisms proposed to be involved. The terms *light* and *deep* sleep refer to

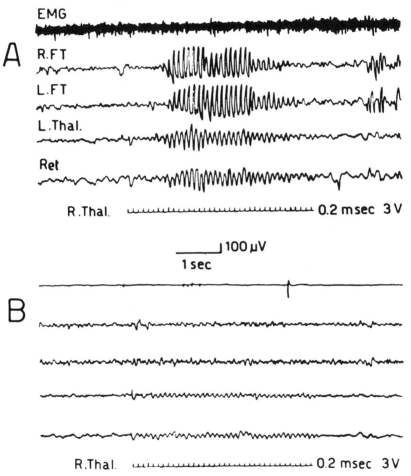

Fig. 99. Records of EMG and electrical activity of cortex, thalamus and midbrain reticular formation, showing large amplitude recruiting responses, induced by low frequency stimulation of intralaminar thalamic nuclei during light sleep (A), and absence of responses to similar stimulation during deep sleep (B). From Rossi *et al.* (1961).

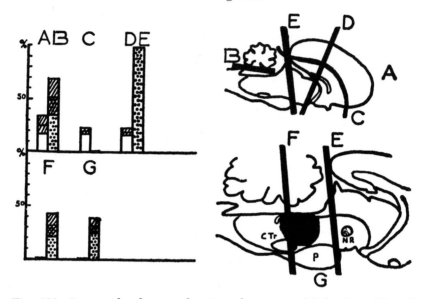

Fig. 100. Bar graphs showing duration of patterns of light (*stipple*) and deep (*white*) sleep, as percentage of twelve hours of continuous recording in cats with neural lesions diagrammed at the right: A. intact, B. cerebellectomized, C. decorticate, D. mesencephalic, E. pontile, F. retropontile and G. medial lesions of pontile reticular formation. Note the absence of light sleep after decortication (C) and the absence of deep sleep after retropontile (F) or medial pontile (G) lesions. Obviously, the cortical EEG is not influenced during deep sleep in mesencephalic and pontile cats. Deep sleep is distinguished, in these preparations, by changes in pontile electrical activity and in the EMG. From Jouvet (1961).

the increased difficulty in awakening the sleeping animal by peripheral afferent or direct reticular stimulation during deep, as compared with light sleep. The terms *slow-wave* and *fast-wave* (or activated) sleep refer to the patterns of electrocortical activity which characterize the two stages. The term *paradoxical* sleep refers to the surprising resemblance between the EEG pattern of deep sleep and that of wakefulness.

It seems possible to make a synthesis of these several designations, and additionally to relate them to the presence or absence of subjective dreaming, if emphasis is placed upon the parts of the brain which undergo inhibition during each stage of sleep, rather than upon the site of the inhibiting mechanisms, or other features. It can be proposed that in the light, slow-wave stage of sleep, cortical function is predominantly impaired. In this stage, synchronization of the cortical EEG may be the consequence of prolonged repolarizing and hyperpolarizing post-synaptic potentials, blocking the spontaneous activity of the non-specific thalamo-cortical projection system and rendering it un-responsive to excitatory drives (Purpura, Cohen and Shofer, 1962). These changes, in turn, may contribute to gating other neuronal discharge into ineffective firing patterns (Calma and Arduini, 1954). Arousal from this stage of sleep is relatively easy, for other subcortical mechanisms are predominantly un-involved. Subjective dreaming is lacking for the pronounced EEG synchronization would appear to provide a substrate of cortical function inadequate to support subjective experience.

Contrastingly, it can be proposed that in the deep, fast-wave stage of sleep, subcortical function is predominantly impaired. The absence of slow waves in the electrocortical record is attrib-utable to inhibition of the nonspecific thalamo-cortical synchro-nizing mechanism, which is no longer excitable, even to direct stimulation. Arousal from this stage is difficult, because of in-hibition of the ascending reticular activating system. As noted, much higher than usual intensities of afferent or direct reticular stimulation are necessary to induce general wakefulness in this deep stage of sleep. The paradoxical pattern of EEG arousal, characteristic of this deep stage of sleep, appears adequate to sup-port degrees of subjective experience, including intense emotion, in dreaming. The pronounced limbic hypersynchrony observed during deep sleep suggests that differences in hippocampal activ-ity may be of great significance here, and perhaps especially so in relation to memory-processing and the exceedingly brief period of recall, usually associated with dreaming. The lack of motor manifestations, except for eye movements and occasional twitch-ing of face or limbs, during dreaming, may be attributed either to inhibition of the reticulo-spinal facilitatory system or, con-versely, to excitation of the bulbar reticulo-spinal system capable of widespread inhibition of lower motor activity.

More generally, it has long been known that varying degrees of wakefulness exist and, from these exciting recent advances, it is no longer possible to consider sleep a unitary behavior. From current work, two stages of sleep can be differentiated: by distinctive patterns of electro-cortical activity, by different levels of arousability, and by the presence or absence of dreaming. The degree of involvement of somato-vegetative alterations is also distinctive. These categories of light, slow-wave and of deep, activated sleep, can seemingly be attributed respectively to the inhibition of predominantly cortical, and of predominantly subcortical levels of the brain.

REFERENCES

Calma, I. and Arduini, A.: Spontaneous and induced activity in pyramidal units. *J. Neurophysiol.*, *17*:321-335, 1954.

Dement, W.: The occurrence of low voltage, fast EEG patterns during behavioral sleep in the cat. *EEG Clin. Neurophysiol.*, *10*:291-296, 1958.

Dement, W.: The effect of dream deprivation. *Science*, *131*:1705-1707, 1960.

Dement, W. and Kleitman, N.: Cyclic variations of EEG during sleep and their relation to eye movements, body motility and dreaming. *EEG Clin. Neurophysiol.*, 9:673-690, 1957.

Hara, T., Favale, E., Rossi, G. F. and Sacco, G.: Richerche sull'attivita elettrica cerebrale durante il sonno nel gatto. *Riv. Neurol.*, *30*:448-460, 1960.

Hubel, D. H.: Electrocorticograms in cats during natural sleep. *Arch. ital. Biol.*, 98:171-181, 1960.

Jouvet, M.: Telencephalic and rhombencephalic sleep in the cat, pp. 188-208. In Wolstenholme, G. E. W. and O'Connor, M. (Eds.) *The Nature of Sleep*, Churchill, London, 1961.

Jouvet, M.: Recherches sur les structures nerveuses et les mecanismes responsables des differentes phases du sommeil physiologique. *Arch. ital. Biol.*, *100*:125-206, 1962.

Kleitman, N.: The nature of dreaming, pp. 349-374. In Wolstenholme, G. E. W. and O'Connor, M. (Eds.) *The Nature of Sleep*, Churchill, London, 1961.

Purpura, D. P., Cohen, B. and Shofer, R.: Activities of thalamic neurons during evoked EEG synchronization and activation. *Trans. Am. Neurol. Assoc.*, 1962.

Rossi, G. F., Favale, E., Hara, T., Giussani, A. and Sacco, G.: Researches on the nervous mechanisms underlying deep sleep in the cat. *Arch. ital. Biol.*, 99:270-292, 1961.

11

CONCLUSION

When one attempts to formulate generalizations concerning the developments discussed above, and to characterize their additions to the rich contributions of the Edwardian period, the introduction of a more operational point of view both in neuronal and brain function seems to form the most obtrusive feature.

Within the individual neuron, graded response mechanisms have been identified at each end of the classically conducting nerve fiber. These have greatly increased the scope of comprehension of neuronal function over that provided by the concept of all-or-none activity now confined to the conducting axon.

Within the brain, a central transactional core has been identified between the strictly sensory or motor systems of classical neurology. This central reticular mechanism has been found capable of grading the activity of most other parts of the brain. It does this as a reflection of its own internal excitability, in turn a consequence of both afferent and corticifugal neural influences, as well as of the titer of circulating transmitters and hormones which affect and modify reticular activity.

While the functions of this reticular system tend generally to be more widespread than those of the specific systems of the brain, it is proposed to be subdivided into a grosser and more tonically operating component in the lower brain stem, subserving global alterations in excitability, as distinguished from a more cephalic, thalamic component with greater capacities for fractionated, shifting influences upon focal regions of the brain.

Influences of this reticular system which are directed spinalward modify the activities of motor outflows from the cord, in particular those subserving postural control. Reticular influences which are directed forward to the cephalic brain stem and limbic forebrain, affect mechanisms regulating visceral and endocrine functions, as well as innate and emotional behavior.

In its ascending and descending relations with the cerebral cortex, the reticular system is intimately bound up with, and contributes to most categories of higher nervous activity. It has to do significantly with the initiation and maintenance of wakefulness; with the orienting reflex and focus of attention; with sensory control processes including habituation and external inhibition; with conditional learning; through its functional relations with the hippocampus and temporal cortex, with memory functions; and, through its relations with the midline thalamus and pontile tegmentum, with the management of internal inhibition, as well as light and deep sleep. These manifold and varied capacities of the reticular system suggest that it serves importantly and in the closest conjuncion with the cortex in most of the central integrative processes of the brain.

Chaucer (Parlement of Foules, l. 22) once remarked, "For out of old fields, as men saithe, cometh all the new corn, fro yere to yere." Hopefully, all the new corn reported here will in some degree advance current understanding of the relations of brain function, on the one hand—to behavior and, on the other—to the mind.